Hand Splinting
Principles of Design and Fabrication

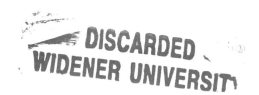

Hand Splinting
Principles of Design and Fabrication

JUDITH C WILTON

MS PGradDipHlthSc BAppSc(OT)

Hand Therapist, Hand Rehabilitation Specialists, Perth, Western Australia;
Coordinator Post Graduate Diploma in Hand and Upper Limb Rehabilitation,
Curtin University of Technology, Perth, Western Australia

with contributions from

TERRI A DIVAL

BAppSc(OT)

Hand Therapist, Hand Rehabilitation Specialists,
Perth, Western Australia.

WB Saunders Company Ltd

London • Philadelphia • Toronto • Sydney • Tokyo

WB Saunders Company Ltd   24–28 Oval Road
London NW1 7DX

The Curtis Center
Independence Square West
Philadelphia, PA 19106–3399, USA

Harcourt Brace & Company
55 Horner Avenue
Toronto, Ontario M8Z 4X6, Canada

Harcourt Brace & Company, Australia
30–52 Smidmore Street
Marrickville, NSW 2204, Australia

Harcourt Brace & Company, Japan
Ichibancho Central Building, 22–1 Ichibancho
Chiyoda-ku, Tokyo 102, Japan

© 1997 WB Saunders Company Ltd

This book is printed on acid free paper

A catalogue record for this book is available from the British Library

ISBN 0-7020-2214-4

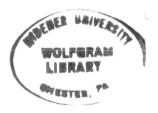

Typeset by J&L Composition Ltd, Filey, North Yorkshire

Printed and bound at the Bath Press, Avon, UK.

Contents

Contents

Preface

Hand Splinting: Principles of Design and Fabrication is intended to be a very practical book for occupational and physiotherapy practitioners and students who do not have extensive knowledge or experience in splinting the elbow, forearm and hand. Splinting is primarily used in the management of trauma, diseases affecting musculoskeletal systems, principally arthritis, and central nervous system dysfunction. It will be assumed that the reader has a basic understanding of anatomy, physiology and pathology pertinent to these conditions.

The book is divided into four sections. The first section contains three chapters of theoretical and technical information essential to prescription, design and manufacture of upper limb splints. Chapter 1 focuses on clinical reasoning to assist the therapist to determine the role of splinting in optimizing hand function for a given patient or client. The functions of a splint – to immobilize mobilize, or restrict – are discussed in relation to healing and disease processes, and the requirements for occupational performance. Chapter 2 addresses the biomechanical principles that pertain to the design of splints while Chapter 3 provides more technical information about materials, equipment and resources used to manufacture a splint.

The second section contains four chapters that address regional splinting in the elbow and forearm, the wrist and hand, the fingers and the thumb for the conditions of trauma and arthritis. In each of these chapters the anatomy is discussed. This is by no means a comprehensive coverage but rather highlights specific anatomical features pertinent to splinting intervention. Splints are discussed according to their function with one or two splints identified for more detailed information as to their design and fabrication procedure. It is the desire of the authors that the basic pattern-making and fabrication skills will form the building blocks for competency in design and manufacture of more complex splints. It is recommended that these chapters are not read in isolation from the first section.

The third section addresses splinting and casting in the presence of central nervous system dysfunction. The need for a specific chapter arises in part from the complexity of issues associated with splinting this population and the fact that splinting is not the usual domain of the neurological therapist. It addresses the traditional methods of splinting and casting, and introduces the developments in use of Lycra® as a dynamic splinting medium.

In the last section, four case studies are used to synthesize material from preceding chapters. Clinical reasoning is based upon foundations of information. This chapter aims to provide some of the building blocks to that foundation. It attempts to put the human face to the problems confronting the patient and his or her therapist. The case studies are discussed from differing perspectives to demonstrate clinical reasoning issues pertinent to splint prescription and manufacture.

Whilst many diagnostic specific splints are described in the literature, it is not the intention of this book to address splint design and fabrication from this premise. Therefore, there are no 'splinting protocols'. Many excellent books exist which address the therapeutic processes involved in the management of specific diagnoses.

In therapy circles, focus is directed to the splint product, however, fabrication of a quality splint is only a small part of the total process. Confident application of splinting materials to injured or painful hands comes with practice. No skill, whether it be creating a piece of furniture or hitting a golf ball, becomes more accomplished without practice. Splinting is a therapeutic modality that can achieve some very specific therapeutic goals. Unlike many other aspects of therapy, the evidence of intervention is worn by the client outside the therapy environment. Therefore, the quality of intervention, the competence of the therapist, and his or her skills in prescription, design and fabrication can be judged by the patient, the family, the medical team and others.

Judith Wilton

Acknowledgements

This book is a result of years of clinical practice where patients have used their knowledge and experience to challenge my foundations of splint design and fabrication, and years of educating undergraduates and graduate therapists who continue to teach me ways to facilitate development of their knowledge and skills, whilst avoiding many of the 'minefields' present in splinting practice. To past and present patients and students 'thank you'.

To Terri Dival a very special 'thank you' for her wonderful support as a friend and colleague, and for her excellent contribution to this book. To Stephen, Lorin and Lucas, thank you for allowing Terri the time and space to contribute to this book, and for being there when we needed you!

My appreciation is also extended to Bill Bassett-Scarfe for his patience and perseverance in getting the illustrations 'just right'; to Jenni Ballantyne for providing information and illustrations on lycra splints; to Nancy Ferris for her assistance in pattern design; to Ray Dival, David Bryant, and Max Heinrich for their critical review and constructive advice regarding content of the biomechanics chapter; to Dr Lee Neylon for his constructive comments on the biomechanics and anatomy sections; to Marion White and Ross Wilton for their diligence and perseverance over many hours of editorial review; and to Miranda Bromage and staff at WB Saunders for their expertise in making this book a reality.

Finally, to my family and friends a very big 'thank you' for their understanding and support throughout the writing of this book.

Judith Wilton

Glossary of Terms

Actuating force – dynamic force that produces movement and allows movement.

Client – a person with a lifelong disability who receives therapy intervention which does not relate to an acute illness or exacerbation of disease.

Contracture – persistent loss of full passive range of motion at a joint resulting from structural changes in connective tissues.

Force arm – the part of a lever between the axis and the point of application of force.

High-profile dynamic splint – the dynamic traction is applied directly to the outrigger. The outrigger thus sits high above the limb to accommodate the required length in the vertical traction.

Lever – a rigid structure which imparts pressure or motion from a force at one point against a resisting force at another point to cause movement or resist movement occurring at an axis of motion.

Low-profile dynamic splint – the outrigger is low, sitting close to the limb to serve as a pulley for the dynamic traction unit. Traction is passed through the outrigger and then travels horizontally to attach more proximally on the splint base.

Manipulatory force – force which produces a counterforce to oppose gravity, tissue tension or muscle action, to position, prevent movement or restrict movement.

Moment – torque.

Moment arm – the perpendicular distance from the line of application of force to the axis of rotation.

Moment of force – torque.

Patient – a person receiving treatment for an acute illness or exacerbation of disease within a medical model of practice.

Pressure – compression force which is applied perpendicularly to the skin. Total force per unit area of application.

Reactive force – a force applied to ensure the effect of the primary force applied is directed to the desired target.

Resistance arm – the part of a lever between the axis and the point of application of resistance.

Rotational force – the component of an applied force which resolves into a purely rotational effect. That component which is resolved to being applied at 90° to the lever being acted on.

Shear stress – compression forces which are applied tangentially (at an angle) across the surface of the skin with a rotational effect on the tissue.

Spasticity – 'a motor disorder characterized by a velocity dependent increase in tonic stretch reflexes (muscle tone)' (Young and Weigner, 1987, pp. 50).

Stabilizing force – force applied to stabilize and secure a splint on the limb.

Torque – the rotational effect of a force.

Translational force – the component of an applied force which resolves into a compressive or distracting force.

Reference

Young R R, Wiegner A W [1987] Spasticity. *Clinical Orthopaedics and Related Research.* **219**: 50–62.

1

Splint Prescription: Clinical Reasoning Issues

Introduction
•
Assessment for Splinting Intervention
•
The Purpose of Splinting
•
Functions of a Splint
•
Patient Issues Pertinent to Splint Design and Fabrication
•
Conclusion

Introduction

Rehabilitation of the hand is one of the significant challenges for therapists working with persons with disease or trauma affecting the upper limb. Hands, and hand function, are such a vital and demonstrative part of one's body and personality that impairment or disability has serious implications for emotional well-being and performance of occupational tasks. Restoration of, or maximizing potential for, optimum hand function is a common objective of therapy intervention. Hand splinting is an integral part of this intervention.

Clinical reasoning is the thinking and decision-making process associated with clinical practice. The theoretical information that must be synthesized prior to making a decision about the use of splinting as an integral part of a therapy regime is extensive. It includes:

1. Knowledge of pathology, anatomy and kinesiology so that the problem presented by the patient can be identified.
2. Knowledge of the procedures and practice of therapeutic intervention of which splinting is but one modality.
3. Knowledge of the purposes, functions and principles of splint design and fabrication.
4. Technical skills and knowledge of splint fabrication procedures.

The development of clinical expertise requires knowledge and skill to be used in the context of practice where the unique characteristics of the patient will influence decisions made by the therapist. In addition, the culture in which the practice occurs will also determine the course of intervention. Factors such as health policy, medical hierarchy and economics have to be considered.

The focus of this chapter is to provide information that will assist a therapist to determine the role of splinting in achieving objectives to optimize hand function for a given patient or client. Issues pertinent to problem identification are discussed prior to identifying the purposes and functions of a splint. The last section focuses on the patients and their characteristics which will impact on the prescribed treatment.

Assessment for Splinting Intervention

Whilst many patients are referred to therapy 'for a splint', the therapist should acknowledge that the patient has been referred for 'therapy', which, in the opinion of the referring doctor or surgeon, should include the application of a splint. As with any other form of therapeutic intervention, an evaluation is required. The process and instruments selected by the therapist are determined by the patient, the diagnosis and the information required.

In the acute phases of injury or disease, the therapist is concerned with the tissues involved in the pathology. Knowledge of the mechanism of injury, the surgical intervention and duration from onset of pathology will assist in determining the degree of tissue integrity, the response of tissues to the injury, surgery or disease process,

and the stage of the healing process. Function of the hand is evaluated at the level of impairment with determination of joint motion, muscle strength, sensory status, level of amputation and severity of pain experienced. Good communication between the referring doctor and the therapist will ensure all relevant information is gleaned prior to commencing intervention. This is essential for the formulation of a treatment plan, including the choice of media and modalities. Splinting is one therapeutic modality that can achieve some very specific goals, but it is rarely an intervention in isolation.

In less acute stages of injury or disease, the focus of assessment changes from the various tissues of the upper limb, to the accomplishment of tasks undertaken by the patient using the affected limb. Instruments that scrutinize hand function at this level attempt to quantify or describe disability. Disability of the upper limb can not be assessed with one instrument as the demands that a person places on the hand and arm may vary from fine coordination and dexterity to considerable power and endurance. Many instruments are described in the literature to assess performance in activities of daily living, object manipulation, tool use and work capacity. Whilst the primary goal of hand rehabilitation is to optimize the patient's ability to function in their environment, it is essential that assessment is undertaken to ascertain whether the splint prescribed facilitates or hinders this objective.

Irrespective of the level of hand function assessed, instruments provide information to identify the need for patient treatment, to evaluate progress of dysfunction or outcome of intervention, to compare the patient's hand function status to the norm, and as a basis of professional communication and accountability. However, the quality of the information gathered is determined by the reliability, validity and sensitivity of evaluation instruments used.

On completion of the evaluation, the therapist will have identified a number of problems. The next stage in the therapeutic process involves prioritizing these and identifying the most appropriate therapeutic interventions to address each problem. Splinting may be the media of choice. One splint may address several problems, or in some instances several splints may be designed and fabricated. As the patient progresses in rehabilitation, obviously the problems will change along with the objectives and types of splinting intervention.

The process of assessment, which identifies a potential role for splints in achieving the therapeutic objective, must also identify precautions and contraindications. Precautions in the use of splinting as a therapeutic intervention pertain to the integrity and sensibility of the skin, and the viability of the peripheral vascular system, irrespective of the diagnosis.

The Purpose of Splinting

Splinting intervention may be used to:

1. Immobilize, stabilize or protect tissues in the acute phases of wound healing following injury, surgery or exacerbation of disease.
2. Immobilize, stabilize or protect tissues when their integrity has been compromised by chronic disease.
3. Protect tissues that are at risk of deformity and contracture subsequent to paralysis or altered muscle tone.
4. Optimize functional use of the upper limb.

5. Substitute for paralysed musculature.
6. Correct deformity.

Functions of a Splint

Identifying that the patient requires a splint as an integral part of the treatment process presupposes a knowledge of the purpose and functions of a splint. Immobilization, mobilization and restriction are identified as the key functions a splint can perform on a body part (American Society of Hand Therapists' Splint Classification System, 1992). Prescription of a splint or splints with one or more of these functions will fulfil the medical requirements for tissue management and the objectives of the patient for recovery of optimal function. This section will consider the key issues pertaining to selection of splint function to resolve identified problems in the upper limb. Descriptions of individual splints that fulfil these functions are discussed in later chapters.

Splinting to Immobilize Tissues

When using static splints to stop joint motion and thus immobilize tissues, there is a distinction between those that immobilize tissues to facilitate wound healing and those that allow the tissues to rest in optimal positions to limit pain or support paralysed musculature. The differences pertain to the position of immobilization, and to the duration and frequency of splint application.

IMMOBILIZATION FOR REST

The normal resting position adopted by the hand is determined by the bony architecture, capsular length, and the length and resting tone of the

3

intrinsic and extrinsic muscles of the wrist and hand. The wrist is generally positioned between 10° and 20° extension with minimal ulnar deviation, the finger metacarpophalangeal (MCP) joints in 20°–40° flexion, and the finger interphalangeal (IP) joints 0°–15° flexion. The thumb is slightly abducted at the carpometacarpal (CMC) joint, and in a few degrees of flexion at the MCP and IP joints. Splints designed to rest tissues should adopt a similar position for immobilization (Figure 1). Following injury, or exacerbation of disease, the hand assumes a posture determined by the impact of pathology on the normal tension within the wrist and hand musculature, the degree of swelling in the wrist and hand, and the integrity of the bony, capsular and ligamentous structures. The tendency is for wrist flexion and ulnar deviation, finger MCP joint extension, proximal interphalangeal (PIP) joint flexion greater than 45° and slight distal interphalangeal (DIP) joint flexion. The thumb is slightly abducted and extended to a position just lateral to the index finger. This position flattens the normal longitudinal and transverse arches found in the hand, in addition to altering the arches of the thumb. In the presence of paralysis, adoption of this posture will result in significant compromise of function should contracture result and then re-innervation occur or reconstructive surgery be attempted (Figure 2). Regaining motion secondary to contracture associated with this position is most difficult in abduction of the thumb, flexion of the finger MCP joints, extension of the PIP joints and flexion of the DIP joints.

The positions of immobilization of the hand achieved by splinting aim to maintain normal anatomical relationships. Deformity is commonly seen following joint and tissue destruction associated with arthritic diseases. Altered biomechanics of the muscles entrench certain positions

Figure 1 Immobilization of the wrist and hand in a position of rest.

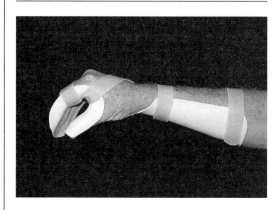

Figure 2 Resting posture of the hand with long-standing paralysis secondary to an incomplete spinal cord lesion at C5.

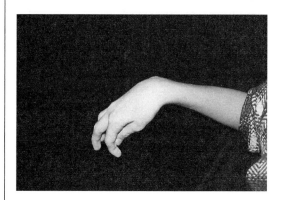

that may lead to contracture of tissues. Gentle correction of a deformity, whilst immobilized in a resting splint, can provide pain relief and prevent permanent shortening of tissues. Splints that immobilize the hand in the presence of paralysis, or diseases with permanent deformity, are worn for extended periods of time, and thus should position the hand to minimize possible complications associated with loss of length and flexibility of capsular structures and muscle tendon units. Further discussion on immobilization of specific parts of the hand is found in subsequent chapters.

IMMOBILIZATION TO FACILITATE THE WOUND-HEALING PROCESS

A knowledge of the responses of tissue to injury and the physiology of the subsequent wound-healing process is the basis for clinical decision-making in hand and upper limb rehabilitation. It is also the basis for splint design and application. Wound repair, as characterized by the three phases of inflammation, fibroplasia, and remodelling, is well described in the literature. The major issue with application to splint design and fabrication is that of wound strength.

Surgical repair to restore the association of structures can provide stability through various pins, plates, screws and external fixation devices in the case of bone, and strength from suture materials in the case of connective tissues and skin. Immobilization by casts and splints is a common method used to provide external strength or stability until the tissues have regained sufficient strength to withstand the normal stresses associated with their function. Where immobilization is required following injury or surgery, the position required, along with the duration of immobilization, is determined by the specific pathology of the tissues involved. Thus good communication with the surgeon is necessary.

In the presence of acute inflammation, whether from trauma, surgery or infection, the immediate vascular and cellular response is designed to destroy bacteria and clear the tissue space of dead and dying cells so that repair processes can begin. The wound is predominantly cellular, with little inherent strength, owing to lysis of collagen within and at the margins of the wound. The increase in tensile strength that takes place during the fibroplastic phase, beginning 2–5 days post-injury, corresponds to increasing amounts of collagen in the wound. This phase consists of fibro-plastic proliferation and capillary growth as a result of cell migration and proliferation. During this period, immobilization helps prevent collagen fibre and capillary disruption, and facilitates the increase in tensile strength of the wound (Peacock, 1983).

Collagen content increases rapidly for approximately 3 weeks at which time it reaches a plateau as a result of balancing rates of collagen degradation and synthesis. At this time the wound is a single unit with newly synthesized collagen tissue invading all aspects of the wound. Whilst this has advantages for re-establishing integrity and strength, it has serious implications to the free gliding of mobile structures. This 'one wound' concept as described by Peacock (1983) results in adhesions between skin and tendon, and tendon and bone that have the potential to limit motion severely. Re-establishment of a gliding function requires motion and stress to be applied to the tissues, so that randomly orientated collagen fibrils uniting all injured structures during the early phase of the healing, become orientated to a structure resembling the pre-injury state. Splinting is thus often combined with other movement modalities designed to gain differential glide between tissue structures. A progressive increase in tensile strength of the wound continues for up to a year.

Wound contraction is an important aspect of the fibroplastic phase designed to close a wound in which there has been loss of tissue (Peacock, 1983). Whilst multiple theories abound as to the process of wound contraction (Rudolph et al., 1992), manipulation of wound contraction remains primarily mechanical via surgery, or the use of splints or casts to maintain tissues in a lengthened position. Where there is sufficient tissue mobility, contraction is not a problem, however, deformity may occur if the wound crosses a concave or joint surface. A possible end result of the process of contraction is a deficit in passive range of motion, flexibility and/or differential glide of tissues. Scar contracture is a result of the contractile process occurring in a healed wound and often results in an undesirable, fixed rigid scar causing deformity (Rudolph *et al.*, 1992).

Where wound contraction is a significant risk, as in the case of burns, the position in which the hand is immobilized in the splint becomes critical. The 'position of safe immobilization', a term coined by Boscheinen-Morrin *et al.* (1992), considers the relative length of capsular structures of the MCP, PIP and DIP joints in addition to the ultimate functional demands of the hand requiring length and extensibility of the dorsal skin of the hand.

Splinting tissues to minimize the complications associated with wound contraction are quite specific to the location of the wound and the tissues involved (Figure 3). When instigating a therapy programme that addresses this issue, it is important that all tissues are considered. For example, it

might be ideal to maintain the hand in an extended position to maintain full length of palmar skin following palmar burns and skin grafting; however, this position will compromise the length of capsular structures of the MCP joints. Thus the clinical decision-making of the therapist demands synthesis of pathology and anatomy to plan a splinting programme that addresses the unique requirements of the tissues for an optimum healing environment, without compromise of the ultimate functional result.

As the strength of the wound increases, the need for continued immobilization declines. The duration of immobilization of injured tissues is directly related to their inherent strength and function. For example, skin grafts are immobilized for 3–5 days whilst bone fractures are immobilized up to 6 weeks. The maturation or remodelling phase may last for many months. Tensile strength progressively increases with approximately 50% of normal tensile strength regained by 6 weeks (Smith, 1995). At this stage the objective of splinting intervention may change from immobilization to mobilization.

IMMOBILIZATION TO FACILITATE FUNCTION

Splints that immobilize joints whilst facilitating functional use of the hand generally address the thumb and/or wrist. Rarely are fingers immobilized. Immobilization of an unstable or painful joint in the position of function commonly used by the patient can increase the potential for involvement of the hand and upper limb in self-care, vocational or avocational activities. The position of immobilization should be determined in consultation with the patient as dominant and non-dominant hands often have different functional

Figure 3   Position of immobilization of this hand with dorsal burns maintains joint capsular structures and skin connective tissues in a position which minimizes risks of contracture.

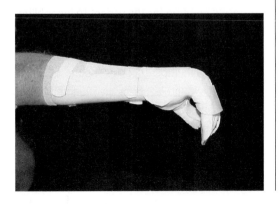

Table 1
Positions of Immobilization of the Wrist and Hand

Joint	Resting position	Safe position (in relation to capsular structures)	Functional range[1]
Wrist	10°–20° extension	Neutral–10° extension	15°–40° extension
Finger MCP	20°–30° flexion	greater than 45° flexion	15°–70° flexion
Finger PIP	0°–20° flexion	0°–10° flexion	0°–60° flexion
Finger DIP	Slight flexion	0°–10° flexion	20°–40° flexion
Thumb	Slightly extended and abducted at CMC with slight flexion of MCP and IP	Abduction extension Rotation at CMC Extension of MCP and IP	Abduction and opposition at CMC with slight flexion of MCP and IP

[1] Angle of immobilization will be determined by the patient's requirements in performance of occupational tasks.

requirements. Table 1 provides a summary of positions for immobilization of the wrist and hand.

CONSEQUENCES OF PROLONGED IMMOBILIZATION

The dilemma commonly faced by therapists and surgeons is to protect injured structures long enough to allow them to repair, yet mobilize them early enough to avoid the complications of immobilization and/or scarring. Restriction in the range of motion of a joint is fundamental to the development of contracture. This restriction may arise from pain, joint destruction or incongruity, wound contraction, immobilization imposed by a cast or splint, neurological disorders affecting muscle function or, indeed, a combination of several factors.

The effects of immobilization on tissues are well documented (Akeson *et al.*, 1980, 1987, Donatelli and Owens-Burkhart, 1981). Akeson *et al.* (1987) summarize the changes in synovial joints as:

- Proliferation of fibro fatty connective tissue within the joint space that adheres to the cartilage surfaces.

- Formation of adhesions between the folds of the synovial lining.
- Atrophy of the cartilage.
- Disorganization of the cellular and fibrillar arrangement of the ligaments, and their attachment to the bone.
- Generalized osteoporosis of cancellous and cortical bone.

The response of skeletal muscle to immobilization is atrophy with a significant decrease in the rate of protein synthesis and adaptation to immobilized position with changes in the number and length of sarcomeres (Tabary *et al.*, 1972; Williams and Goldspink, 1978).

It is not uncommon for the patient to immobilize the injured part and, in severe cases, the whole upper limb. When pain is combined with fear complete immobilization of the limb results.

Immobilization of tissues in any splint carries some significant responsibilities for the therapist. The benefits of joint rest in terms of pain relief, decreased inflammation, or increasing potential healing must be weighed against the possible adverse functional deficits that may

Figure 4   Joint contracture in the position of immobilization and chronic oedema are the consequences of poor splint design.

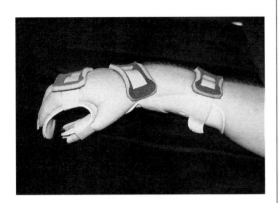

Figure 5   Regaining length and extensibility in the thumb index web, and in wrist extension, is the purpose of this splint worn by a patient with severe fractures of the distal radius and ulna.

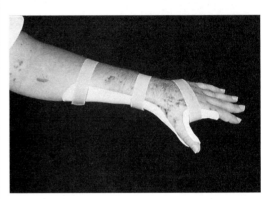

arise secondary to disuse and contracture. Figure 4 illustrates the consequences of poor splinting to rest a hand with pain associated with reflex sympathetic dystrophy.

Splinting to Mobilize Tissue

Mobilization splints are designed to remodel tissue according to its functional requirements of length and extensibility, or to substitute for paralysed or spastic musculature. Therefore, careful assessment of the muscular and connective tissues will identify whether the deficit in motion is active (owing to weakness or paralysis of musculature), passive (owing to connective tissue limitations) or a combination of both. The literature identifies three types of mobilizing splints (Fess, 1987; Colditz, 1995).

TYPES OF MOBILIZING SPLINTS

Serial static splints (and casts) Whilst static in nature, serial static splints are described as mobilizing splints because they are designed to mobilize or lengthen tissues. They are moulded in one position at the end range of the elastic limit of tissues (Figure 5). A period of time is allowed for tissues to respond to the position prior to the splint being remoulded, or cast replaced, in the new lengthened position. Serial splints or casts maximize the time tissues are maintained at end range as they are generally worn for periods of between 10 and 24 hours per day.

Serial casts or splints are used for moderate to severe joint contractures (Bell-Krotoski, 1995) and for deficits in muscle tendon unit length (Tribuzi, 1995). In the presence of pain and chronic inflammation, sustained force applied by serial static splints is generally tolerated better than the intermittent stress applied by dynamic splints (Colditz, 1995). The disadvantages of serial casting or splinting are the loss of active motion in the direction opposite the contracture and risks associated with immobilization.

Dynamic splints Regardless of their design or purpose, dynamic splints 'create a mobilizing force on a segment, resulting in passive or passive assisted motion of a joint or successive joints'

Figure 6   Dynamic splint with elastic traction applied to the finger middle phalanx in the directions of flexion and extension.

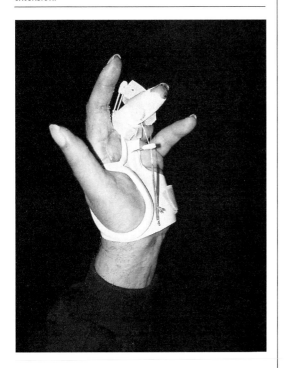

Figure 7   A hinge at the elbow allows the range of elbow motion to be progressively increased as tissues respond.

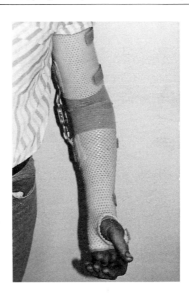

(Fess, 1987, p. 86). Splints designed to increase passive range of motion create their forces through elastic bands, springs or mechanical devices (Figure 6), whilst dynamic Lycra® splints use the elastic properties within the fabric to create their force. The dynamic component continues to apply force when the tissues reach their maximum length. Therefore, the size of force applied is critical as too much can cause trauma to the tissue and result in an inflammatory response. Thus splints are applied intermittently as tolerance to sustained force of this nature is generally not greater than several hours.

In the presence of paralysis, dynamic splints redirect active motion of non-paralysed muscles to effect motion in target joints. A common example is the use of tenodesis action where wrist motion is coupled with finger motion.

Static progressive splints These splints are similar to dynamic splints in construction and design. However, the mobilizing force is created by non-dynamic components such as Velcro®, hinges, screws or turnbuckles (Figure 7). The tissues are positioned at the end range of their elastic limit for a period of time prior to adjustment of the joint position as the passive range of motion (PROM) changes. Advantages of this type of splint are twofold. Firstly, the mobilizing force remains constant for a given application at the predetermined joint range and, secondly, active muscle contraction against the mobilizing force is not possible, thereby maximizing the time spent at the end of the available joint range.

PRINCIPLES OF APPLICATION OF MOBILIZING SPLINTS TO ADDRESS DEFICITS IN JOINT RANGE OF MOTION

Tissue response to stress Mobilizing splints are used to correct deformity through application of gentle forces, resulting in an increase in passive range of joint motion. In order to apply stress safely to resolve joint contracture, an understanding of soft tissue response to stress is required. Brand and Thompson (1992) and Brody (1986) describe four phases in the lengthening response of tissues. The initial phase, where internal elements of the tissues unfold, is followed by gradual alignment of internal elements with the primary stresses. Stiffening of tissue elements occurs when all elements are aligned with the stress. Further incremental increase in stress results in smaller and smaller amounts of lengthening until ultimate failure is caused by internal disruption of the tissue (Figure 8).

When the force used stretches tissues beyond their normal elastic limit, microscopic tears of fibres and cells may cause an inflammatory reaction. This inflammation may cause fibrinogen to be laid down resulting in an even greater limitation in motion. Where failure or disruption of tissues has not occurred, their response to unloading will be determined by the nature of the tissue, the proportion of elastic versus inelastic components and the length of time the force was applied. Recovery of shape and dimension on removal of the force is described as elastic deformation, whilst retention of length and shape is due to the viscous nature of tissues demonstrating plastic deformation.

When safe forces are applied to tissues, either statically or cyclically, they demonstrate a transient lengthening depending upon viscoelastic properties of the tissues. Brand and Thompson (1992) note that elongation of tissue accompanied by stretch will shorten again once the force is relaxed. The lengthening that occurs within 24–48 hours is creep. Creep is the lengthening that occurs in material held under constant load over time. Growth occurs over weeks and is associated with the normal turnover of tissue. Thus remodelling in tissues held in a lengthened position, for a period of hours or days, ultimately depends on the ability of the cells to sense and transduce the mechanical force into biological action and grow (Arem and Madden, 1976).

In the clinical setting, measurement of torque range of motion has been used to determine the mechanical quality of tissues that limit joint motion. This measurement is recommended prior to determining the appropriate splinting intervention for stiff joints (Fess and Philips, 1987; Brand and Hollister, 1992; Schultz-Johnson, 1992; Bell-Krotoski, 1995). Torque range of motion is the method of measuring a joint with a standard goniometer whilst a known force is used to position the joint. 'Starting at the joint's resting position, higher and higher torques are applied until the joint's end range is reached.' (Flowers and Pheasant, 1988, p. 69). The torque angle curve, as illustrated in Figure 9, is the graphic representation of these measurements.

A gentle curve is characteristic of compliant tissues with a 'soft end feel' whilst a steep curve is characteristic of non-compliant tissues with dense parallel collagen fibres and thus a 'hard

Figure 8   Soft tissue response to applied tension. Phase: 1, unfolding; 2, alignment; 3, stiffening; 4, failure.

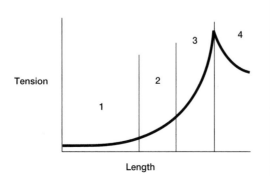

Figure 9   Graph of torque angle measurements for two interphalangeal finger joints.

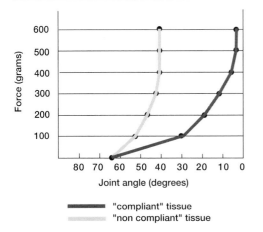

"compliant" tissue
"non compliant" tissue

end feel' to joint motion. It is suggested that: gentle curves have a good prognosis with dynamic splinting; steep curves require static or static progressive splinting; and very steep curves are more likely to require surgery to resolve the contracture. These recommendations are based on laboratory studies of tissue responses to stress. However, Prosser (1996) in a study of 20 persons with stiff PIP joints, found no direct association between torque angle curve and ultimate resolution of contracture following treatment with dynamic splinting. Experience would suggest that the time of splint application has more influence on resolution of contractures with either a soft or hard end feel than splint design.

Intensity and timing of force application Factors critical in the resolution of deficits in joint range of motion are the time of initial application, and the intensity and duration of force applied. When deficits in range of motion exist, a splinting programme will minimize long-term deformity. This is achieved by gently influencing the laying down of collagen fibres during the fibroplasia and early remodelling phases of wound healing. The timing of the initial application of stress is crucial as stress applied too early post-injury may prolong the inflammatory response. Greater caution is required where tissues have not stabilized and fluctuation in oedema still occurs.

The total stress used to modify contracture is a product of the tension, or compression, and the time it is applied to the tissues. McClure (1994) suggests that therapists consider total stress applied to the tissues as a 'dose' of treatment. An insufficient dose of stress will have no therapeutic effect, while an excessive dose may produce complications such as pain and inflammation.

Brand and Hollister (1992) encourage the use of a gentle force for a prolonged period of time to effect permanent changes in length of tissues. The principle of low-load prolonged stress is accepted as the premise of mobilizing splinting. However, the quantity of force required to mobilize a deficit in range of motion (ROM) remains unclear. Commonly recommended forces of 100–300 g (Fess and Phillips, 1987; Brand and Hollister, 1992) are based upon the skin and the subcutaneous tissue tolerance to pressure and not the rotational effect of the stress on the actual contracted tissues. Rotational effect or torque is the product of the stress and the distance from the axis on which the stress is applied. The suggestion by Fess and Philips (1987) that the force should be lowered if it is applied further from the axis of the joint assumes tissue pressure tolerance approximates the torque stress tolerated by the contracted tissues. Further discussion of these principles is undertaken in Chapter 2.

Kottke *et al.* (1966) investigated the association between time and intensity of force application in addressing chronic joint contractures. They found that prolonged stretching at moderate tension produced significantly greater restoration of motion, within the limits of pain and without evidence of tissue tearing, than did intense stretching of short duration. Time of splint wearing appears to be the primary factor associated with the resolution of joint contracture.

Little empirical evidence exists to provide guides to the most appropriate duration of splinting in terms of hours per day and days per year in order to resolve tissue contracture. Kolumban (1969) suggested 8–11 hours per day over an extended time. Watson and Turkeltaub (1988) and Snell and Connolly (1989) recommend splinting of 3 months duration. Prosser (1996) in a study of 20 persons with PIP joint contractures observed that between 65% and 90% of the improvement in joint range was achieved within the first 2 weeks of wearing a dynamic splint for between 6 and 14 hours per day. The balance of improvement occurred over a period of 3–5 months.

Flowers and Michlovitz (1988) introduced the term 'total end range time' (TERT) to focus attention on the summation of all the time the joint is held at end range to stimulate growth of tissue. Splint application has significant potential to maximize TERT over other forms of intervention. For example, if a mobilizing splint is worn for 2 hours per day, TERT is 2 hours in the 24 hours available, and 14 hours in the 168 hours available over a week. Alternatively, if joint mobilization techniques are applied for 20 minutes per joint per working day, the TERT is 20 minutes in 1440 minutes per day and 2.5 hours in 168 hours per week. Therefore, a mobilizing splint is more effective in maximizing TERT than other forms of therapeutic mobilization.

Experience has shown that patients will generally tolerate static progressive splints for longer per-iods than dynamic splints. In addition, stress to mobilize hand tissues in the direction of extension is tolerated for longer periods than stress in the direction of flexion.

When choosing the time to apply mobilizing splints, the therapist must consider the patient's requirements for functional hand use, the application of therapeutic modalities other than splinting and, in some cases, the number of splints incorporated into the programme. Sleep affords the hand an extended period of rest each day and is often an ideal time to apply splints. Without the demands for functional use, the hand may be splinted for extended periods of uninterrupted time. Prior to application at night, it is important to ensure there are no problems from extended wear during waking hours. It is also important to ensure components such as traction can not be inadvertently altered by bedding or poor positioning.

Cessation of splinting intervention is appropriate when the deficit in passive ROM is resolved and can be maintained by active motion. If a contracture has not resolved but gains in passive ROM have plateaued, gradual weaning from the splint is appropriate. The exception is where active range of motion does not sustain passive gains. Intermittent periods of wear may continue, generally at night so that function is not impaired, until stabilization of the wound-healing process has occurred. Remodelling of tissue can occur for many months and discarding splints prior to maturation of the scar tissue is unwise. In some cases this may mean splints are worn for several hours per day for many months.

Precautions to application of mobilizing splints Exacerbation of pain and swelling may be indicators of problems arising from application of mobilizing splints. Some discomfort is not uncommon when the mobilizing force is first removed from the tissues; however, persistence of pain and discomfort, directly attributable to splinting, for periods longer than 10 minutes is indicative that the dose of stress was too great. In this situation reduction in the force and/or reduction in the time of application are necessary. If the use of dynamic splints, with intermittent application of stress, is the cause of problems, consideration should also be given to application of continuous stress by serial static and serial progressive splints.

MOBILIZING SPLINTS TO ADDRESS PARALYSIS AND SPASTICITY

In the presence of paralysis, without joint contracture, splints can redirect active motion of non-paralysed muscles to effect motion in target joints. The unique coupling of the wrist and finger musculature in the tenodesis action allows a therapist to design splints to facilitate grip and pinch function. The action of the wrist musculature can be harnessed to approximate the fingers to the thumb for pinch, or to extend the fingers for reach. These splints are effective for specific movements with wearing schedules determined by the patient's function activities. In the presence of paralysis, splints are worn until recovery of function occurs by either reinnervation or tendon transfer.

The use of custom-made dynamic Lycra® splints (Figure 10) to facilitate functional movements in the presence of upper limb spasticity is a relatively new innovation. Where dominant patterns of spasticity are coupled with weakness in the antagonist muscles, severe restrictions in patterns of grasp and release exist. Lycra® splints use the inherent properties of the Lycra®, that is the desire to recover from its elastic deformation, to

Figure 10 The usual typing posture (a), determined by spasticity in the wrist and finger musculature, of this client with cerebral palsy is slow and tiring. A dynamic lycra splint (b) addresses the position of the wrist and fingers to facilitate more efficient use of the hand.

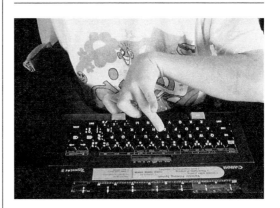

a

b

resist the spastic muscle action, while also facilitating the antagonist action to achieve a predetermined functional goal.

Splinting to Restrict the Function of Tissues

Restriction splints are those that limit a specific aspect of joint range of motion. Restriction of joint motion is used to provide an optimum environment for wound healing and to facilitate functional use of the limb.

RESTRICTION OF TISSUES TO FACILITATE HEALING

Tissues in the hand glide in relation to each other to permit intricate complex movements essential to function. Injury to one structure or system in the hand is rare. Therefore, the interrelationship between intrinsic and extrinsic structures requiring different excursion will be affected if complete immobilization of the hand is undertaken in order to allow one or several structures to heal. Maintenance of gliding will only happen if controlled motion is allowed, minimizing the possibility of one wound resulting in one scar. Studies have shown that early motion increases the tensile strength in repaired tendons (Gelberman *et al.*, 1983) and speeds repair of cartilage (Salter *et al.*, 1980). Splints used following tendon repairs fall into this category. Finger or thumb movement is restricted in one range of motion so that undue stress is not placed on the tendon repairs. Secondary joints, such as the wrist, are commonly immobilized.

RESTRICTION OF TISSUES TO FACILITATE FUNCTION

Following peripheral nerve palsy, restriction of motion in one joint may allow movement to be redirected to movements in other joints thus facilitating function of the hand. For example, following ulnar nerve palsy, if MCP joint extension is restricted, the extensor digitorum communis (EDC) tendons can effect PIP and DIP extension and flexor digitorum profundus (FDP) and flexor digitorum superficialis (FDS) can flex the fingers towards the palm for effective grasp. Similarly, restricting the motion of the joint to prevent instability or pain at extremes of movement will also increase functional potential.

Problems associated with rigidity, compromise of some aspects of hand function and the discom-fort from splints made of thermoplastic materials has led to increased availability of a wide range of 'soft' splints. Custom made and prefabricated splints in elastic, neoprene or leather materials provide tissue constraint and support whilst restricting some motion.

Splinting to Facilitate Function

Many splints manufactured specifically to facilitate functional use of the hand may be classified within the categories of immobilization, mobilization or restriction. However, there is a group of splints designed to facilitate a particular functional task that do not fit these categories. Splints designed to hold a pen, pencil or an eating utensil, to allow control in driving a car, or to isolate a digit to facilitate computer access are commonly used in the presence of permanent paralysis or dysfunction.

Patient Issues Pertinent to Splint Design and Fabrication

In the majority of therapeutic interventions used to address musculoskeletal dysfunction, the therapist has direct control of the procedure. However, splinting is one intervention where the patient or his or her carer has the control. The bottom line to successful splinting intervention is that the patient must wear the splint if it is to achieve its objectives. Consideration of factors unique to the patient, his or her attitudes, lifestyle, and living and working environment, will increase the potential for an optimal outcome. Interactive reasoning, based on face to face communication between the therapist and the patient, will directly influence many aspects of splint design. Failure to consider the unique aspects of the patient and his or her lifestyle may jeopardize the success of the very best splint.

Patient Responsibility in Splinting Intervention

Immediately following an acute injury, decisions regarding the splint design, the splinting material and the wearing regime are generally made by the therapist or surgeon, with minimal contribution from the patient. In many instances no choice is offered as the patient is either too sick, or has no experience or foundation upon which to make any decisions about splinting intervention. The nature of the injury determines the splint requirements.

In the presence of chronic dysfunction, however, the patient has more extensive experience with hand dysfunction and often splinting, so may identify specific splint requirements. A clear explanation as to the purpose for splinting intervention, the reasons and rationale for the design, the wearing regime and precautions, should be discussed prior to the patient making a decision that splint fabrication should proceed.

Studies undertaken on compliance to splinting persons with chronic hand dysfunction suggest it varies between 25% and 65% (Belcon et al., 1984). The literature suggests compliance to splinting intervention is greater when:

- The benefits of the intervention are immediately obvious (Nicholas et al., 1982; Hicks, 1985; Groth and Wulf, 1995). ˙
- The patient's family supports the intervention (Oakes et al., 1970).
- The therapist provides education to the patient of the benefits of the splint and expected wearing regime (Nicholas et al., 1982; Feinberg, 1992).

- The therapist affirms his or her belief in the positive benefits of splinting intervention for the patient (Law et al., 1991; Feinberg, 1992).

For those patients who are very young, very sick, who have altered levels of consciousness or an intellectual impairment, or who are unable to communicate their response to intervention, the therapist must assume the responsibility for safe application of splints. The therapist must involve parents, relatives or those responsible for the patient's care in decisions regarding splinting intervention. Education of carers and implementation of strategies that monitor intervention are essential to minimize risk of injury.

Age

Age is also a strong determinant of the type and design of splint intervention.

CHILDREN

For very young children, the challenge is to maximize the effects of splinting within the context of the child's intelligence and tolerance to intervention. Issues of co-operation during splint fabrication can be addressed by establishing the parent's and child's confidence in the process, by having a non-threatening splinting environment where tools and the heating pan are not in direct view of the child, by allowing the child to play with the splinting material and perhaps splint a favourite toy (Figure 11) or a parent prior to fabrication. It is important to mould the splint right on the first attempt as distressing the child will not facilitate a positive attitude to the splint, splint wearing or returning to therapy. Burns, from heated thermoplastic materials and hot water, are a very real risk when splinting very young children. Ideally, splinting materials should have a low activation

Figure 11 A wrist immobilization splint for both child and doll. Other decorative features were added later by the mother.

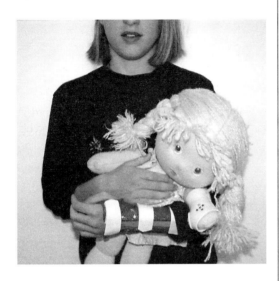

Figure 12 A post-operative splint for a 17-month-old baby has volar and dorsal components for the hand and forearm, and includes the elbow for anchorage.

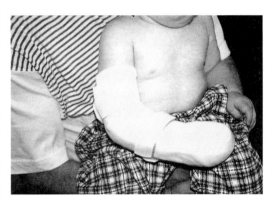

temperature, a quick set-up time and a memory, or the ability to be remoulded several times to accommodate for growth.

Design features specific to children often require the following.

1. Inclusion of more proximal joints to anchor the splint Splints need to be more extensive where they are required to protect structures post-operatively to eliminate risks of further injury during play. Incorporation of the elbow to anchor a splint to the arm is not uncommon (Figure 12). Risks associated with immobilization of uninvolved joints and structures are minimal in this age group.

2. Use of circumferential designs to gain strength and ensure good pressure dispersion over very fragile skin Circumferential splint designs made of lighter thinner materials (1.6 mm) use contour to gain strength, disperse pressure and eliminate any risks of straps being applied too tightly.

Baby and toddler skin, with its subcutaneous fat, do not tolerate straps wells. All straps should be wide and contour to the area applied. Fabrication of a 'tough' splint, that is not too heavy or cumbersome, yet able to protect structures during play, will alleviate some of the fears of parents and reduce restrictions necessary for children during splint wear.

3. An effective means to secure the splint to the limb Laced ties and buttons combined with Velcro® may be necessary to impede ingenious and inquisitive little people removing splints during unsupervised periods of wear. A splint may also be held in place by self-adhesive bandage such as Coban or a crepe bandage secured by tape. A sock or stocking cover will also provide some degree of protection against the splint injuring another body part following spontaneous arm movements.

4. Incorporation of features that facilitate compliance to wearing Special features applicable to the child's age and interests may be incorporated into the splint. The use of coloured splinting materials, trims in sporting team colours, decorative transfers or disguises in the form of gloves or puppets, should assist compliance to wearing. However, it is important that features applied to increase compliance do not detract from the use of functional hand splints.

Parents and carers of children have a unique role in ensuring compliance to splint wearing, therefore, they should contribute to the decision-making processes associated with design and fabrication.

ADOLESCENTS

Compliance to splint intervention is a major consideration when addressing deformity and dysfunction in the hand of adolescent patients with permanent conditions such as rheumatoid arthritis or cerebral palsy. In this age group, body image is particularly important and, therefore, any form of splinting intervention must also fit into this schema. Logical reasoning by the therapist based on long-term gains will not necessarily win out over short-term acceptance within a peer group. The first step in the splinting process is for the patient to make an informed decision that a splint will address his or her specific need. The second step is for the therapist to ensure the aesthetic appearance is acceptable to the patient. The final step is to determine a wearing schedule that is sensitive to the patient's lifestyle whilst still achieving the specific requirements of the intervention.

ELDERLY

Issues pertaining to splinting the elderly are centred on the fragility of the skin and its ability to tolerate stress. With little subcutaneous fat and a slowed healing response, consideration must be given to meeting the objectives for splinting intervention whilst being fully aware of the risks of loss in function or injury from a splint. Where toughness of skin is not maintained by normal func-

tional use of the hand, it becomes very soft and vulnerable to breakdown. In a fisted hand, the lack of airflow around the fingers and thumb maintains a warm moist environment that increases the risks of bacterial and fungal infection. Choice of materials is critical. Perforated splinting materials and washable lining materials are recommended.

Cognitive status is also a critical issue. Clear written instructions, to assist both the patient and his or her carer, are often required to accommodate diminished memory and a confused state of mind. Acceptance of change is often difficult for the elderly person, so gradual introduction to splint wearing may be necessary in non-acute situations. Modified straps and closures for splints may also be necessary for those persons with dementia.

It is recommended that the focus of assessment for splinting intervention goes beyond the hand and upper limb, as many elderly patients have a complex medical history. Whilst the medical problem may not be the focus of splinting intervention, it may have a direct impact on the design and fabrication. A common example is diabetes, where design features may change in the presence of compromised peripheral circulation and sensibility.

Environment and Lifestyle Factors

Consideration of the environment in which the splint will be worn will identify those persons who will assume responsibility for application of the splint. In an acute setting, such as a burns unit, it may be the nursing staff, in a school setting, it may be a teacher's aide, but in the majority of cases it will be the splint wearer. Experience suggests that persons who contribute to the decision-making process, who are well informed as to the purpose of splinting intervention and who are convinced that the therapist believes the splint will achieve its objectives are more likely to be compliant. Attitudinal and motivational factors impact upon compliance, with experience a powerful influence, particularly for patients with a chronic disability.

For those patients who independently manage their own splinting programme, the possible functional impact of wearing a splint on self-care, mobility, vocational and avocational activities should be discussed. Design should maximize independent application and accommodate lifestyle demands. Tolerance to moisture and various chemicals, flexibility, friction to accommodate grip on tools and walking aids in the hand are just some of the factors which impact upon choice of splinting materials.

Musicians and athletes form a unique category of patients, owing to their motivation to return to their vocation early in the phase of healing. This often demands creative splinting designs to address both the therapeutic objectives and the performance requirements of the instrument or sport (Figure 13).

Figure 13   The requirements for immobilization of a fracture and ligamentous injury to the metacarpal of the thumb, and continued functional performance are achieved in a customized splint.

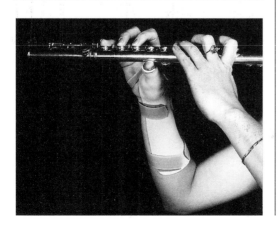

Geographical and Climatic Factors

The geographical location of the patient's home and work will influence the availability for follow-up and indicate the climatic conditions under which the splint will be worn. Many of the splinting protocols which address deficits in range of motion require regular attendance at therapy for modification to the position of the splint, the angle of the outrigger and the force of dynamic traction. If distance prohibits regular attendance, the design must accommodate change without losing effectiveness. Alternatively, education of the patient as to how to modify the splint components to accommodate change is possible in selected cases. In environments where care and maintenance of the splint may be less than ideal, for example, isolated areas such as mining camps, offshore drilling rigs or fishing trawlers, simple serial static splints may be a better choice than complex dynamic splints, owing to the lesser risk of complications of broken or modified components.

Climate will influence the type of splinting and lining materials selected. Comfort is a major factor in compliance to splinting protocols, therefore, the need to use perforated splinting materials where heat and humidity are a major issue will dictate the design options. In the presence of extreme cold, methods to maintain warmth in the hand in the splint should be considered.

Aesthetic Factors

Aesthetic considerations are an important issue for a majority of patients. Consider the person you are making the splint for; their appearance and care associated with their grooming will give some indication of their expectations of a splint.

An important question for all therapists to answer is 'Would I be prepared to wear in public the splint I have just made for my patient?'. Obviously some designs are 'eye-catching' with their function dictating their structure; however, the quality of the finished product provides evidence of the skill and craftsmanship in the design and manufacture. Unless the intent is an unco-ordinated look, the colours of the splinting material, the straps, the finger loops and lining materials should be integrated.

Cost Factors

Cost of therapeutic and splinting intervention is a real consideration for all consumers. Whilst one would wish to provide the best options, may dictate the use of less costly materials for splinting intervention, the use of materials that have a memory and can be remoulded several times, or the use of designs that accommodate several splinting objectives in the one splint. Cost should not compromise design or the objectives of splinting intervention. Prefabricated or commercially made-to-measure splints may be perceived to be more expensive; however, the cost savings in reduced consultation time may warrant their use.

The cost of a splint that fails to meet its objective is extremely high. Both splinting materials and therapist time are expensive; however, the cost incurred by the patient should not be disregarded. When confronted with a problem requiring a complex splint beyond the expertise of the primary therapist, referral to, or consultation with, an experienced therapist competent in splinting can be a cost-effective solution to the problem.

Patient Education

Education of the patient and carers has been shown to increase compliance to therapeutic intervention. Verbal instructions given at the time of fabrication are often forgotten. The event can be quite stressful with the patient coping with a lot of new experiences and a lot of information. Written instructions provide a permanent reminder and allow reference at a later date.

Written instructions should include:

1. A wearing schedule for both day and night.
2. Problems or complications that may arise from wearing a splint.
3. Precautions when wearing the splint.
4. How to care for, clean and maintain the splint.
5. How to contact the therapist should problems arise.
6. A date of review appointment.

Splint-wearing Regimes

Wearing regimes are as variable as diagnoses and patients. In determining an initial or on-going regime the following factors should be considered:

1. The pathology of the effected tissues and acuity of problem.
2. The goal of the splint and, on re-evaluation, its effectiveness in achieving this goal.
3. The patient's lifestyle with specific focus on self-care, vocational and avocational demands of the involved hand.
4. The number of splints in the programme and other therapeutic objectives for active motion and functional performance.

The bottom line to successful intervention is the fact that the patient must wear the splint if it is to achieve its objectives. Therefore, realistic expectations must be set in conjunction with the patient.

Conclusion

Information presented in this chapter underpins clinical reasoning in relation to prescription of splints to address dysfunction in the upper limb. Appropriate splinting intervention is dependent on a sound knowledge of the functions of a splint and the purposes it can achieve. Accurate assessment and determination of the objectives for intervention are the first stages in successful design and fabrication. Whilst the function of the splint may be immobilization, mobilization or restriction of specific joints, the objective may vary widely according to the diagnosis, time from onset of the condition, and the unique qualities of the patient and his or her requirements for function in his or her upper limb.

Splinting the hand and upper limb presents a constant challenge to the therapist as the unique characteristics of the patient combine with their pathology to determine splint requirements. Sensitivity to the patients' needs, their attitudes and lifestyles, and their living and working environments will maximize compliance and will thus increase the potential for an optimal outcome.

References

Akeson, WH, Amiel, D, Abel, M, et al. (1987) Effects of immobilization on joints. *Clinical Orthopaedics & Related Research* **219**: 28–37.

Akeson, W, Amiel, D & Woo, S (1980) Immobility effects on synovial joints: The pathomechanics of joint contracture. *Biorheology* **17**: 95–110.

American Society of Hand Therapists (1992) *Splint Classification System*. Chicago: American Society of Hand Therapists.

Arem, AJ, Madden, JW (1976) Effects of stress on healing wounds: intermittent noncyclical tension. *Journal of Surgical Research* **20**: 275–286.

Bell-Krotoski, JA (1995) Plaster cylinder casting for contractures of the interphalangeal joints. In: Hunter, JM, Makin, EJ, Callahan, AD (eds) *Rehabilitation of the Hand: Surgery and Therapy*, 4th edn, pp. 1609–1616. St Louis: Mosby.

Bell-Krotoski, JA, Breger-Lee, DE, Beach, RB (1995) Biomechanics and evaluation of the hand. In: Hunter, JM, Makin, EJ, Callahan, AD (eds) *Rehabilitation of the Hand: Surgery and Therapy*, 4th edn, pp. 153–184. St Louis: Mosby.

Belcon, MC, Haynes, RB, Tugwell, P (1984) Critical review of compliance studies in rheumatoid arthritis. *Arthritis and Rheumatism* **27**: 1227–1233.

Boscheinen-Morrin, J, Davey, V, Conolly, WB (1992) *The Hand. Fundamentals of Therapy*, 2nd edn, Oxford: Butterworth Heinemann.

Brand, PW, Hollister, A (eds)(1992) *Clinical Mechanics of the Hand*, 2nd edn. St Louis: Mosby.

Brand, P, Thompson, DE (1992) Mechanical resistance. In: Brand, PW, Hollister, A (eds) *Clinical Mechanics of the Hand*, 2nd edn, pp. 92–128. St Louis: CV Mosby.

Brody, GS (1986) The biomechanical properties of tissue. In: Rudolf, R (ed) *Problems in Aesthetic Surgery*, pp. 49–64. St Louis: CV Mosby.

Colditz, JC (1995) Therapists management of the stiff hand. In: Hunter, JM, Makin, EJ, Callahan, AD (eds) *Rehabilitation of the Hand: Surgery and Therapy*, 4th edn, pp. 1141–1159. St Louis: Mosby.

Donatelli, R, Owens-Burkhart, H (1981) Effects of immobilization on the extensibility of periarticular connective tissue. *Journal of Orthopaedic and Sports Physical Therapy* **3**: 67–72.

Feinberg, J (1992) Effect of the arthritis health professional on compliance with use of resting hand splints by patients with rheumatoid arthritis. *Arthritis Care and Research* **5**: 17–23.

Fess, EE, Philips, CA (1987) *Hand Splinting Principles and Methods*, 2nd edn, St Louis: CV Mosby.

Flowers, KR, Michlovitz, SL (1988) Assessment and management of loss of motion in orthopaedic dysfunction. *Post Graduate Advances in Physical Therapy II–VIII*. Alexandria VA: American Physical Therapy Association.

Flowers, KR, Pheasant, SD (1988) The use of torque angle curves in the assessment of digital joint stiffness. *Journal of Hand Therapy* **1**: 69–74.

Gelberman, RH, Vande Berg, JS, Lundberg, GN et al. (1983) Flexor tendon healing and restoration of the gliding surface. *Journal of Bone and Joint Surgery* **65A**: 70–80.

Groth, GN, Wulf, MB (1995) Compliance with hand rehabilitation: health beliefs and strategies. *Journal of Hand Therapy* **8**: 18–22.

Hicks, JE (1985) Compliance: a major factor in the successful treatment of rheumatoid disease. *Comprehensive Therapy* **11**: 31–37.

Kolumban, SL (1969) The role of static and dynamic splints, physiotherapy techniques and time in straightening contractures of the interphalangeal joints. *Leprosy in India*. Oct: 323–328.

Kottke, FJ, Pauley, DL, Ptak, RA (1966) The rationale for prolonged stretching for correction of shortening of connective tissue. *Archives of Physical Medicine and Rehabilitation* **47**: 345–352.

Law, M, Cadman, D, Rosenbaum, P, et al. (1991) Neurodevelopmental therapy and upper-extremity inhibitive casting for children with cerebral palsy. *Developmental Medicine and Child Neurology* **33**: 379–387.

McClure, PW, Blackburn, LG, Dusold, C (1994) The use of splints in the treatment of joint stiffness: Biologic rational and an algorithm for making clinical decisions. *Physical Therapy* **74**: 1101–1107.

Nicholas, JJ, Gruen, H, Weiner, G, *et al.* (1982) Splinting in rheumatoid arthritis: I. Factors affecting patient compliance. *Archives of Physical Medicine and Rehabilitation* **63**: 92–94.

Oakes, TW, Ward, JR, Gray, RM, *et al.* (1970) Family expectations and arthritis patient compliance to hand resting splint regimen. *Journal of Chronic Diseases* **22**: 757–764.

Peacock, EE (1983) Some biochemical and biophysical aspects of joint stiffness: role of collagen synthesis as opposed to altered molecular bonding. *Annals of Surgery* **164**: 1–12.

Prosser, R (1996) Splinting in the management of proximal interphalangeal joint flexion contracture. *Journal of Hand Therapy* **9**: 378–386.

Rudolph, R, Vande Berrg, J, Ehrlich, HP (1992) Wound contraction and scar contracture. In: Cohen, IK, Diegelmann, RF, Lindblad, WJ (eds) *Wound Healing: Biochemical and Clinical Aspects*, pp. 96–114. Philadelphia: WB Saunders Company.

Salter, RB, Simonds, DF, Malcolm, BW, *et al.* (1980) The biological effects of continuous passive motion on the healing of full thickness deficits in articular cartilage: an experimental investigation in the rabbit. *Journal of Bone and Joint Surgery* **62A**: 1232–1251.

Schultz-Johnson, K (1992) Splinting: a problem-solving approach. In:

Stanley, BG, Tribuzi, SM (eds) *Concepts in Hand Rehabilitation*, pp. 238–271. Philadelphia: FA Davis Co.

Smith, KL (1995) Wound care for the hand patient. In: Hunter, JM, Makin, EJ, Callahan, AD (eds) *Rehabilitation of the Hand: Surgery and Therapy*, 4th edn, pp. 237–250. St Louis: Mosby.

Snell, EJ, Connolly, WB (1989) Post-traumatic flexion contracture of the proximal interphalangeal joint, surgical release and post operative therapy — a review of 21 subjects. In *Proceedings of The First Congress of the International Federation of Societies of Hand Therapists*, p. 42. Tel Aviv, Israel.

Tabary, JC, Tabary, C, Tardiue, C, *et al.* G (1972) Physiological and structural changes in the cat's soleus muscle due to immobilization at different lengths by plaster casts. *Journal of Physiology* **224**: 231–244.

Tribuzi, S (1995) Serial plaster splinting. In: Hunter, JM, Makin, EJ, Callahan, AD (eds) *Rehabilitation of the Hand: Surgery and Therapy*, 4th edn, pp. 1599–1608. St Louis: Mosby.

Watson, K, Turkeltaub, S (1988) Stiff joints. In Green, D (ed) *Operative Hand Surgery*, 2nd edn, pp. 537–552. New York: Churchill Livingstone.

Williams, PE, Goldspink, G (1978) Changes in sarcomere length and physiological properties in immobilized muscle. *Journal of Anatomy* **127**: 459–468.

Biomechanical Principles of Design, Fabrication and Application

Introduction
•
Minimization of Pressure
•
Advantageous Application of Forces
•
Advantageous Application of Dynamic Force
•
Utilization of Mechanical Characteristics of Materials
•
Summary

Introduction

'Successful splinting technique is a science firmly based in engineering principle' (Fess, 1995, p. 124). Therefore, an understanding of biomechanical principles is essential to successful design and fabrication of any splint applied to the upper limb. Biomechanics is the unique marriage of physiology and physics that provides sound principles and a simple explanation to successful application of splints. This chapter presents explanations of essential biomechanical principles and their application to splint design and fabrication.

The major biomechanical principles to consider are minimization of pressure, advantageous appli-

cation of forces, advantageous application of dynamic forces and the use of mechanical characteristics of materials. In each section, the concept and its relevance is introduced. Biomechanical analysis explains the theory behind the principle. Clinical implications address those considerations the therapist must think about when applying the principle to the patient and his or her pathology. Clinical applications gives readers a summarized list of rules for the principle that shows how to utilize the information when treating a patient.

The dominant action of all splints is to apply force to the limb with the intent to position, to move or to prevent movement. Force may be considered as compression (push) or tension (pull). Compression is an issue with all types of splints, whilst tension is a critical issue in those splints that use dynamic traction to achieve their effect.

Minimization of Pressure

One of the prime functions of the hand is to apply force to objects in the performance of self-care, vocational and avocational tasks. Tissues are designed to withstand certain amounts of tension and compression and, indeed, the lack of such forces can result in an alteration in histology of bone, cartilage and connective tissues. High force is commonly transmitted through the skin on the volar surface of the hand and often tissues respond by forming a callous. The dorsal surface of the hand rarely has to withstand much force. The skin is thinner with minimal subcutaneous tissue to disperse the force. In the application of force to the hand by a splint, compression forces, and, therefore, pressure, become an issue. Whilst the focus is on the tolerance of skin tissues to external pressure, vascular tissues must also be considered to avoid compromising arterial and venous supply. Some areas, such as the volar forearm, are better able to tolerate pressure than others.

Compression forces may be applied in many directions to the skin. Those applied perpendicularly (generally referred to as *pressure*) are better tolerated than those applied tangentially (at an angle) across the surface of the skin with a rotational effect on the tissue. These directional forces cause what is commonly termed *shear stress*.

When pressure is applied to the skin, a series of events can be observed. There is blanching of the skin due to compression of the microvasculature, and occlusion of the venous return (Thompson, 1995). A change in the contour of the surface also occurs depending upon the type and consistency of subcutaneous tissues. Low stress to the skin of short duration is a normal part of living. However, prolonged low stress to the skin results in displacement of the fluids in the tissues and may eventually change capillary flow and ultimately result in ischaemia. Discomfort and pain can also result from sustained or repetitive pressure. On release of pressure, an area of hyperaemia (redness due to capillary blood flow) may exist.

Fess and Philips (1987, p. 126) state 'a continuous force applied to the extremity should not exceed 50 gm per square centimetre'. However, within the clinical situation measurement of pressure using pressure transducers currently available is not realistic. Discomfort and hyperaemia are signs of pressure being greater than tissue tolerance. Hyperaemia lasting longer than 15 minutes is evidence of inflammation from pressure (Bell-Krotoski *et al.*, 1995).

Repeated pressure has a cumulative effect that may cause a progressive inflammatory change, finally resulting in tissue damage. Brand (1995) demonstrated that tissues that responded to stress with minor inflammatory changes one day required less stress for less time the next day, prior to the same response occurring.

BIOMECHANICAL ANALYSIS

Pressure is defined as force per unit area of application, i.e.

$$\text{Pressure} = \frac{\text{Total force}}{\text{Area of force application}}$$

Therefore, the larger the area over which a predetermined amount of force is applied the smaller the pressure. One hundred grams of force applied to an area of $1\,\text{cm}^2$ equals $100\,\text{g/cm}$ pressure. The same force applied to an area 2 cm^2 equals 50 g/cm pressure. Therefore, when designing a splint, consider the length and width of the splint and its components so that pressure is distributed over a large area (Figure 1). Narrow components of splints, including straps, generally apply higher pressure. Following the contours of the hand will ensure an even pressure distribution between convex areas at high risk (commonly bony prominences) and the periphery of low pressure on concave surfaces (Figure 2).

Shear stress occurs when there are large changes in applied stress, particularly at the interface of the hard splinting material edges and the soft underlying and adjacent tissues. Joint movement, changes in muscle bulk associated with muscle contraction or migration of the splint with movement can also cause shear stress. To minimize shear, the edges of the splint are rolled to ensure a more gradual change in pressure.

Similarly, straps or slings which are not angled to contour to the forearm, hand or finger, can cause shear stress when one edge of the strap or sling lifts away with the sheer stress localized to the

Figure 1   Area of force application. Increase the area of force application to decrease the pressure exerted on the tissue of the forearm. The splint on the left will produce less pressure than the splint on the right.

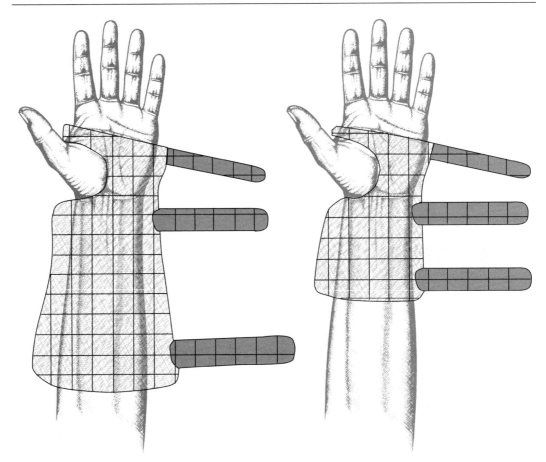

Figure 2 Cross-section through the hand at the proximal palmar crease. The arrows denote areas of potential pressure if the contour of the splint does not equal the contour of the hand.

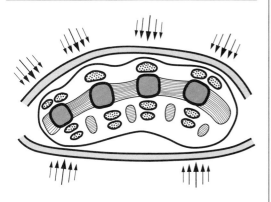

Figure 4 Circulatory compromise from strap pressure. Inattention to presence of pitting oedema has resulted in very obvious circulatory impairment in this patient with reflex sympathetic dystrophy (RSD). Distribution of pressure over the entire surface by uniform circumferential bandaging would have avoided this complication.

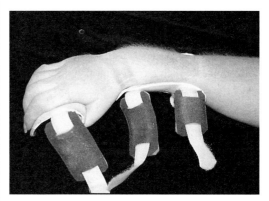

Figure 3 Shear stress with poor strap contour. When the forearm strap is placed on the splint too square, it does not contour to the forearm on closure, causing shear stress at the proximal edge.

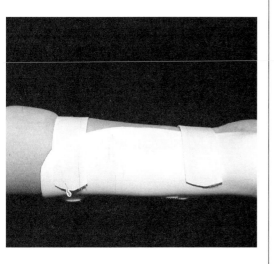

muscle) to disperse the pressure. Particular care is necessary with the dorsum of the hand, the heads of the metacarpals, the radial styloid and the ulnar head to ensure even application of pressure. Identify the potential pressure areas on your own hand. Look closely at your patient's hand as joint disease or injury can significantly alter hand shape and contour.

The therapist must consider the patient's pathology, as conditions that increase fragility of the skin increase the risk of pressure from a splint and thus the potential to cause an injury. Pressure can also compromise vascularity, lymphatic drainage (Figure 4), and sensibility.

CLINICAL APPLICATION

1. Assess tissue tolerance to pressure and shear stress Considering all splints apply pressure, determine the body's ability to tolerate stress. Repeated stress resulting in minor inflammation decreases on subsequent application in normal tissues and, therefore, is of greater concern in the presence of denervation, circulatory

other (Figure 3). The same thing occurs if slings used in dynamic splints no longer pull at 90° (Figure 13).

CLINICAL IMPLICATIONS

Pressure is more critical in those areas of the hand that have minimal subcutaneous tissue (fat or disorders and oedema, fragile skin (as in the case of the elderly or very young), and those persons on steroid therapy or with wounds, grafts or flaps.

It is necessary to ensure no pressure problems exist after an hour of splint wear prior to extended wear. Similarly, application of a low force on dynamic traction, which is subsequently increased with tissue tolerance, is preferable to tissue injury from too great a force.

2. Reduce pressure – increase application area Design splints, including straps, wider and longer to apply less pressure. In situations where anatomy dictates narrow components, acknowledge that pressure may be problematic.

3. Reduce pressure – provide maximum contour Contouring to all skin surfaces increases the area of splint contact and, therefore, increases the area of application of force. All splint components should contour both convex and concave surfaces of the hand to ensure continuous uniform pressure.

4. Reduce pressure – protect areas of risk Padding is not a solution to a pressure problem. Padding that does not bottom out may mimic subcutaneous tissue, and dissipate and absorb some compression force. However, in areas of high risk, such as bony prominences, padding concentrates and, therefore, worsens the risk of pressure. Adding padding over bony prominences only increases the compression by decreasing the space between the tissue and the splint. The solution is to pad out the bony prominence prior to splint fabrication with a small piece of exercise putty moulded over the prominence. If padding is to be used when there are no areas of risk, it is essential that the pad-

ding is incorporated into the design and fabrication, and not added as an afterthought to solve a problem of pressure.

The stabilization of fractures often involves the surgical introduction of external fixation or internal fixation in the form of wires, pins, screws and plates. Particular care is required to avoid pressure between these components and the splint, particularly as post-operative oedema subsides.

5. Reduce shear stress – avoid large sudden changes in pressure The shear effect caused by a sudden change in the pressure gradient at the edge of the splint is reduced by rolling the edges to ensure a more gradual change in pressure. Sheer stress at the edges of straps and slings is avoided by ensuring contour to the limb or digit. Contour is often only achieved by applying straps at an angle (refer to Figure 3).

Advantageous Application of Forces

A splint may be considered as a series of related systems of force application. These force systems are easiest to analyse, apply and remember if described by their intended purpose. This must not be confused with the key functions of immobilization, mobilization or restriction that a splint performs on a body part (as described in Chapter 1).

The types of forces applied by splints to the limb are:

- Stabilizing forces are those forces that are applied to stabilize and secure the splint on the limb.
- Manipulatory forces produce a counterforce to oppose gravity, tissue tension or muscle

action to position, prevent movement or restrict movement.

- Actuating forces are dynamic forces that produce movement and allow movement.

The method of application needs to make the best use of the available force. Inherent in this concept is the notion that the most efficient use of force means using the least energy possible to effect change. The use of minimal force reflects the principles of pressure minimization to protect tissue integrity.

1. Stabilizing Forces

A well-designed stabilizing system prevents migration or rotation of the splint on the limb, avoids zones of pressure concentration by the proximal splint component and maximizes transmission of force by the splint to the targeted tissues. Stabilizing forces provide the base from which manipulatory and actuating forces can effectively be created. They must balance and counteract the forces produced internally by the limb and externally by the distal splint components to produce a system in equilibrium.

2. Manipulatory Forces

The manipulatory forces are those static forces which direct, control or regulate internal and external forces to produce the desired outcome position. In splints that traverse more than one joint, the system must account for movement and position at one joint influencing the movement and position of another.

3. Actuating Forces

Actuating forces require a system to generate dynamic force (e.g. the traction system), a method

of applying or directing this force to the limb (e.g. the outrigger) and a method of attachment of these to the stabilizing splint base.

BIOMECHANICAL ANALYSIS

An understanding of some principles of biomechanics is required at this point. In an effort to create more accessible information, this section will look at the definitions and principles in isolation, remembering in reality the principles are interlinked. The following sections (Clinical Implications and Clinical Applications) will integrate the information.

1. For every action there is an equal and opposite reaction Newton's third law states that to every action there is always opposed an equal reaction. This is the law of interaction, whereby the mutual actions of two bodies upon each other are always equal and directed to the diametrical parts. Thus, where a body, or body part, a tool or a lever imparts a force to another, the target will impart an equal force back.

2. Leverage A lever is a rigid structure that pivots at a fixed point. It serves to impart pressure or motion from a force applied at one point to a resisting force at another point. It is a tool used to effect movement. In all types of levers there is one or more activating force, one or more resistive force, and an axis around which these two sets of forces are applied. The lever itself consists of a fulcrum or axis (the pivot point), a force arm (that part between the axis and the applied force) and a resistance arm (that part between the axis and the resistance). In splinting, the axis is generally the joint the splint is designed to influence. The resistance is the part of the limb to which manipulatory or actuating forces are directed, and the force is the stabilizing, manipulatory or actuating force created by the splint.

For simplicity, levers are classified as first class, second class or third class, depending on the configuration of the force, axis and resistance (Figure 5), but it should be remembered this is

---

Figure 5   Classification of levers. x = axis; a = force; b = resistance; f.a. = force arm; r.a. = resistance arm. Solid arrows denote direction of force application; broken arrows denote potential direction of movement. (a) The first class lever has the axis situated between the force and the resistance. The simplest example is the playground see-saw or teeter-totter. With the axis at x, a force must be applied at a to counteract the weight or resistance at b. If the force applied at a is greater than the resistance applied at b, movement will occur in the direction indicated by the dotted arrow. If the resistance applied at b is greater, the dashed arrow indicates the direction of movement. (b) The second class lever has the resistance between the axis and the force. The wheelbarrow is an example of a second class lever. (c) The third class lever has the force applied between the resistance and the axis. The fishing rod is an example of the third class lever. Concentric action of most muscles in the body is of a third class lever.

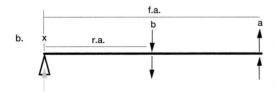

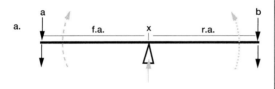

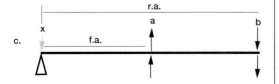

purely arbitrary. It is only intended to make analysis of force and mechanical advantage less complicated and should not be the source of pedantic analysis. The same action often can variously be described as a first, second or third class lever, depending on what point is chosen as the axis. The essential element is that all forces and their associated distances are considered in the analysis.

In a well-fabricated static splint, the forces will always be directed perpendicularly to the longitudinal axis of the body part to be influenced. Resolution of forces is not addressed at this point, but is discussed later in the chapter under Advantageous Application of Dynamic Force.

The designation of a force does not indicate whether it 'pushes' or 'pulls' at the lever. It is the quantity, point of application and the direction of application that is important. In any lever, there must be clockwise and counterclockwise forces around the axis.

3. Systems in equilibrium In any leverage situation, the system is said to be in equilibrium when the sum of the clockwise rotational forces equals and balances the sum of the counterclockwise rotational forces and there is no resultant movement about the axis. These forces are calculated by the equation:

Force × force arm = Resistance × resistance arm

$$f \times f.a. = r \times r.a.$$

i.e. Force torque = Resistance torque

Forces can be applied at any angle to a lever. The force refers to the rotary or perpendicular component of the applied force (refer to Resolution of Forces). The length quantity (f.a. and r.a.) is the distance between the axis and the point of application of force. Where there is force or resistance applied over the whole length of the force or resistance arm, which is usual in static splints, the centre of gravity of the lever arm is the point designated to measure length. If the rotary effects are equal, the lever will not move. If one is greater than the other, there will be resultant movement about the axis.

4. Mechanical advantage

$$\text{Mechanical advantage} = \frac{\text{Force arm}}{\text{Resistance arm}}$$

The function of a lever is to produce more efficient work. The intent is to create a mechanical advantage to effect the desired output. The longer the force arm, then the greater the mechanical advantage. A long resistance arm signifies mechanical disadvantage (Figures 6 and 7).

5. Direction of force application

Many splints applied in the clinical setting utilize three points of pressure arranged in a linear pattern to control or effect joint motion. The middle force is generally directed opposite to the proximal and distal forces (Fess, 1995). Generally, one force is directed to targeted tissues to maintain a position or to increase joint range (Figure 8). The balance of forces is used to control other joints, so that the force is not dissipated by unwanted motion of the more mobile joints or migration of the splint with associated shear forces. Circumferential splints use circumferential forces directed inward to a central point and so have no opposing middle force.

In order for the application of force to result in a desired motion or maintenance of position, a reactive force must be applied to ensure the potential work is directed to the target joint axis. Without these reactive forces, unwanted movement will occur, such as motion at joints

Figure 6   Mechanical advantage. x = joint axis; a, b, c = positions of force application. Increasing the length of the proximal component of a wrist splint increases the mechanical advantage.

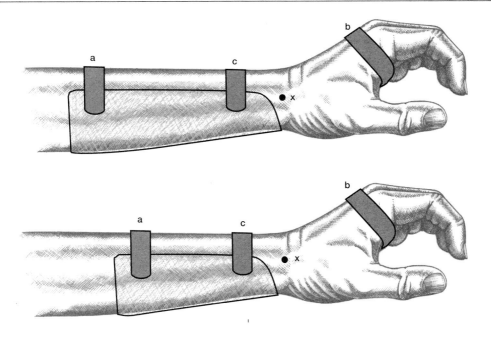

TA Dival, JC Wilton

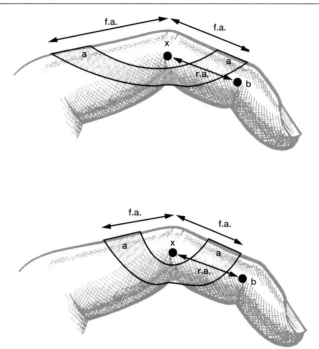

Figure 7 Mechanical advantage. x = joint axis of proximal interphalangeal (PIP) joint; a = position of force application; b = joint axis of distal interphalangeal (DIP) joint; f.a. = force arm; r.a. = resistance arm. In a splint to restrict extension of the PIP joint, the proximal and distal components provide the forces to resist the extension force applied through the resistance arm. By lengthening the force arms, less force is required through a to maintain a position of flexion.

proximal or distal to the target, or rotation around an undesired axis (see Figure 13). The system in its entirety must be analysed to determine the most appropriate and the most effective placement of forces.

Another view of application of forces is the concept of force couples. Force couples produce rotary motion around a point or axis of rotation by acting in opposing directions at separate points around the axis. In dynamic pronation–supination splints (see Figure 14 of Chapter 4), forces are applied in opposite linear directions but in the same direction of rotation.

6. Torque Torque is defined as the rotational effect of a mechanism. The terms 'moment' or 'moment of force' are also used interchangeably with torque. Torque is the product of the applied force multiplied by the perpendicular distance from the axis of rotation to the line of application of the force.

Torque = force × distance

The perpendicular (i.e. shortest) distance from the axis to the line of application of the force is described as the moment arm (Figure 9).

There are three methods to maximize torque:

- Apply greater force.
- Apply force further from the axis.
- Apply force perpendicular to the lever.

When a force is applied to a lever arm at 90°, the moment arm is equal to the force arm (Figure 9a). The total magnitude of the force is applied as a

Figure 8   Direction of force application. x = joint axis; a, b, c = position and direction of force application. In order to effect motion or position at the targeted tissues at x, force needs to be applied in the directions designated at a, b and c.

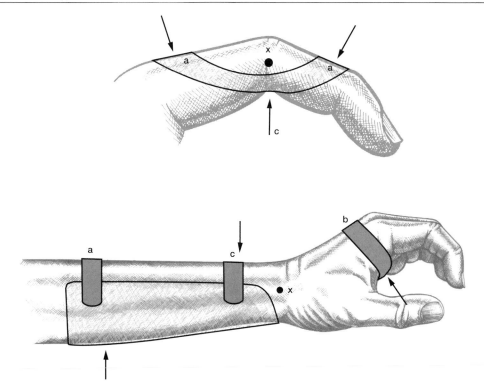

rotational action. Where a force is applied at greater or less than 90°, the moment arm is shortened (Figures 9b and c) and consequently torque is reduced. Where the angle of application is less than 90°, in the resolution of force some of the applied force is lost as a compressive force (Figure 9b). If the angle of application is greater than 90°, some of the applied force is lost as a distracting force (Figure 9c). Therefore, to create optimal rotational force, force must be applied as close to perpendicular to the lever as possible.

There are two methods to calculate torque, using the formula $T = f \times d$:

1. 'F' is the actual applied force and 'd' is the calculated moment arm of the distance between the axis and the line of application of the force.

2. 'D' is the actual distance between the axis and the point of application of the force and 'f' is the calculated resultant rotational vector when the actual force is resolved.

Both methods produce the same result, but the former is usually easier to carry out.

7. Pulley action A pulley provides a method of changing the direction of a force to improve its angle of application. It allows a force generated from any means and position to be redirected to the desired target to produce movement in the desired direction or to increase effective rotational force.

Figure 9 Resolution of forces. When force is applied to a limb part, it may produce a number of effects on the axis (the joint). With a force designed to extend the PIP joint, the force arm being acted on is the longitudinal axis of the middle phalanx between the PIP joint axis and the point of application of the sling. When the traction force is applied perpendicular to the force arm (a), the length of the moment arm equals the length of the force arm. When the actual force of traction is applied at less than (b) or greater than (c) 90°, the moment arm no longer equals the force arm, but is shorter. The traction force is partially resolved into rotational effect and partially into translational force.

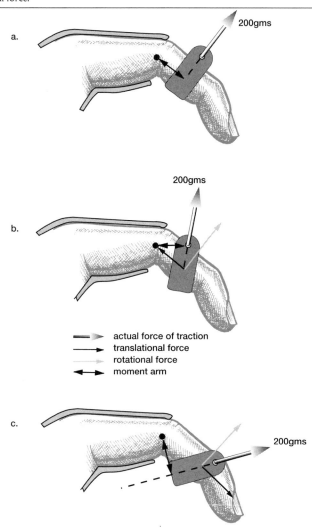

CLINICAL IMPLICATIONS

The therapist must integrate knowledge from a range of sciences to enable him or her to formulate a logical, comprehensive and complete method of designing the most beneficial splint. The difficulty for therapists, particularly students, novices and those who splint intermittently, is to remember all essential aspects of anatomy, kinesiology, biomechanics, pathology and physiology. This section explains a method, or process of thought, which can be followed to integrate and utilize the previously presented information to design a successful splint.

1. Identify the splint purpose Utilizing information from Chapter 1, determine which is the desired function of the splint – immobilization, mobilization or restriction. Determine if one splint can achieve the desired purpose.

2. Identify the forces required to achieve the splint function Identify what manipulatory forces are required and to which joints or tissues they should be directed. Determine whether any actuating forces are required and to which tissues they must be directed.

3. Identify appropriate force placement Utilizing concepts of direction of force application, determine the most effective placement of forces. Consider first the manipulatory and actuating forces and then the required stabilizing forces. Using anatomical, kinesiological and functional knowledge, evaluate how the forces are to be applied. Are they to be applied to volar or dorsal surfaces? Are palmar bars, or dorsal or volar restriction required? Is circumferential force required or can straps apply the required force? The wrist immobilization splint demonstrates this dilemma. The choice to achieve this position includes volar, dorsal, dorsal–volar or circumferential designs.

Generally, if a splint is to impact on a joint, it must traverse it. However, the splint may impact on intrinsic forces within the limb which may affect tissues not directly influenced by splint forces. For example, tension in multi-joint muscles may influence joints proximal or distal to the applied splint forces. These effects may need to be controlled or, indeed, may be beneficially utilized by the splint forces to achieve the desired outcome.

4. Design the application of manipulatory forces The application of manipulatory forces should be considered as a lever system, where the axis is the axis of the joint on which the therapist wishes to impact. The resistance is the part of the limb that must be positioned and the force is applied by the splint in opposition to the weight or action of that part.

Using principles of mechanical advantage, the longer the force arm, the greater the advantage. The length is restricted only by the necessity to protect anatomical function. For example, movement of joints distal to the splint must not be compromised.

Principles of minimization of pressure must be addressed. As the length of the force arm at best will still only approximate the length of the resistance arm, large force will be exerted between the force arm (the splint) and the resistance arm (the limb). That is, there will be large compression forces on the tissues of the limb. In order to minimize pressure, the force should be distributed over the largest possible area.

Principles of torque and the optimization of rotational force should be applied by providing correct contour to ensure the force is directed at 90° to the resistance arm (see Figure 8).

5. Design the application of actuating forces The application of actuating forces is concerned with gaining optimal rotational force. This is addressed in the following section.

The outrigger and its splint base should be considered a lever system. The axis is the distal point of anchorage to the splint base, the resistance arm is between this point and the sling suspension, and the force arm is the distance between the distal anchorage point and the proximal anchorage point (Figure 10).

Figure 10 Attachment of the outrigger to the splint base. The outrigger and its attachment is a first class lever (axis at x, force arm at x − a, resistance arm at x − b). When the splint is designed with mechanical disadvantage, the downward force at b results in rotation around axis x, and movement in the direction indicated at a.

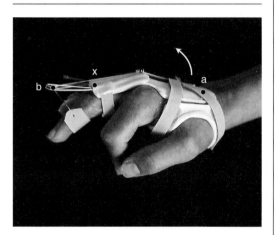

Although some of the resistance force is absorbed by the dynamic component (elastic, spring or coil), there is still significant resistance applied to the resistance arm (the outrigger) by the part being acted upon. This resistance force must be counteracted by an equal force on the force arm (the splint base) to create a system in equilibrium. To create mechanical advantage, the force arm needs to be as long as possible. Where the force arm is short, a system of mechanical disadvantage exists and it is unlikely the outrigger bond or the proximal base will be able to generate enough force to balance the resistance torque. The result is either that the proximal bond fractures or the splint rotates around the lever axis, lifting the proximal base away from hand or forearm. The splint should be designed with the shortest possible resistance arm and the longest possible force arm. There is no mechanical advantage in putting bends in the extension arms of the outrigger. It makes the outrigger more difficult to fabricate and the bends become potential axes of motion i.e. they are a site of potential fatigue.

6. Design the configuration of the stabilizing forces
To impact upon a joint, the splint components must traverse proximal and distal to that joint. This proximal component of the splint gives rise to the required stabilizing forces. By virtue of being approximated to the splint base by some means (commonly a strap), the joint to which the manipulatory or actuating forces are to impact gives rise to a corresponding point on the splint base around which rotary forces are directed. This point becomes the axis of a first class lever. The limb part to which the manipulatory or actuating forces are to be imparted becomes the resistance and the distal manipulatory splint component becomes the resistance arm. The proximal stabilizing splint component becomes the force arm (refer to Figure 8 and translate these lever components to the demonstrated splints).

In order for the system to be in equilibrium, force torque must equal resistance torque. The resistance (the limb), in applying force to the resistance arm, will attempt to rotate the lever around its axis and, in so doing, will rotate the proximal end of the splint, or its stabilizing strap, into the limb. The longer the force arm, the lesser the force applied by the limb to the force arm (the proximal splint) and at the same time a smaller force is applied by the splint to the limb. This becomes an issue of pressure minimization — pressure reduces as the surface area of application increases.

CLINICAL APPLICATION

In summary:

1. Direction of force application has implications for:
   (a) Creating desired rotary motion.
   (b) Preventing undesired motion.
   (c) Directing forces to targeted tissues.

2. Systems in equilibrium have force torque counterbalanced by resistance torque and, therefore, prevent undesired motion.
3. Mechanically advantageous levers maximize the force arm length in relation to the resistance arm length to:
   (a) Minimize force and pressure on tissues.
   (b) Prevent unwanted rotation.
   (c) Prevent component failure and material fatigue.
4. Optimize torque by applying forces at 90° to:
   (a) Maximize the length of the moment arm and ensure the total magnitude of the applied force is converted to rotational force.
   (b) Prevent loss of force to translational force (joint compression or distraction).
   (c) Minimizes shear forces on tissues.
5. Use pulleys to improve the angle of application of force and optimize rotational force.

Advantageous Application of Dynamic Force

Actuating forces are applied by splints by use of dynamic components. These forces produce or allow motion by applying tension to target tissues. Tension is applied to shortened tissues to address deficits in passive range of motion, or tension may be applied to maintain a position at rest from which movement in the opposite direction is allowed or encouraged.

The science of dynamic force application in splinting is still in its infancy. How much force will produce results without risking compromise to tissue integrity or function? How is force measured? How much force actually reaches the targeted tissues? What is the duration (hours per day, days per year) of force application required to effect permanent change?

This section offers a starting point for the therapist, a synopsis of 'where we are now'. The advancement of this science requires further research to enable clinical decisions to be made from more scientific foundations.

Quantification of Force Application

Numerous authors (Fess and Philips, 1987; Brand and Hollister, 1992; Bell-Krotoski et al., 1995) recommend tension forces between 100 and 300 g for the small joints of the hand. However, this figure relates to the compression applied to underlying tissues by the sling or distal splint component, and not the torque applied to the shortened tissues in the vicinity of the joint. The ability of tissue to tolerate this compression is certainly an issue, but critical to clinical efficacy is what quantity of force is translated to joint tissue, and what is the tolerated and beneficial range. Type or classification of tissue is another consideration. It is likely different tissues (ligament, capsule, muscle, tendon, young or old scar) have different beneficial ranges and they respond at different rates to applied forces. Physiological aspects such as vascularity or type and configuration of collagen may also have an influence.

If force is used to elongate tissues beyond their normal elastic limit, microscopic tears of fibres and cells will occur, inducing an inflammatory reaction. Fibrinogen deposition as a result of this inflammation has the potential to create an even greater limitation in motion. More information is needed to determine the safe upper force parameters for tissues. Clinical observation and judgement must be used in the mean time.

There is no literature that provides information on how much torque is required to lengthen a given cross-sectional area of living tissue. To date, discussion has focused on the pressure that can be applied to the skin and subcutaneous tissues, and then translating this into raw force units. However, two splints with the same force applied at different distances from the axis will produce different torques (Figure 11). It is, therefore, torque parameters that must be investigated, not force.

Torque is the rotational effect that is applied to the shortened tissues at the joint. If the same tension

Figure 11   Position of force application. Increasing the distance from the axis at which the force is applied will increase torque.

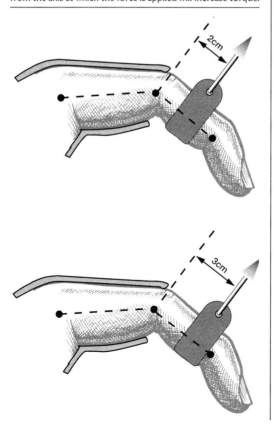

(force) is applied via a sling perpendicular to the lever, the distance from the axis of the joint to the point at which force is applied will determine the torque. For example, 100 g of force applied 2 cm from the axis of the joint will produce 200 Ncm torque. However, if that force is applied 3 cm from the axis of the joint, the torque is 300 Ncm, 150% the original torque. Torque is expressed in Newton centimetres which indicates that both distance and force are critical issues.

Where the force is applied to move a joint through an arc of motion to substitute for paralysed muscle or, in the case of tendon repairs, to substitute for the tendon that needs protection, the force is being applied to 'a passively supple hand' (Fess and Philips, 1987, p. 167). The force applied to the segment need only be sufficient to move the segment to the desired position or alignment.

Resolution of Forces

A tension force applied to a body component may be resolved into two components, the rotational force and the translational force. To maximize the rotational force, the tension must be applied at 90° to the longitudinal axis of the bone distal to the joint being mobilized. In this situation, all the tension is converted to rotational force. When the tension is applied at an angle greater than 90°, some of the rotational force is lost to translational force, which will tend to distract the joint. Similarly, when the tension is applied at an angle less than 90°, some of the rotational force is lost to the translational force, which will tend to compress the joint. This resolution of forces is demonstrated in Figure 9. Therefore, as improvement is made, modifications are required to the outrigger to maintain an appropriate line of pull (Figure 12). The therapist must educate the patient to note the angle of pull and return to the clinic for modification should it not be at 90°.

Figure 12   Modification of angle of force application. As force must be applied at 90° to prevent resolution into translational force, it is critical the application angle of traction force is modified appropriately as the joint contracture resolves.

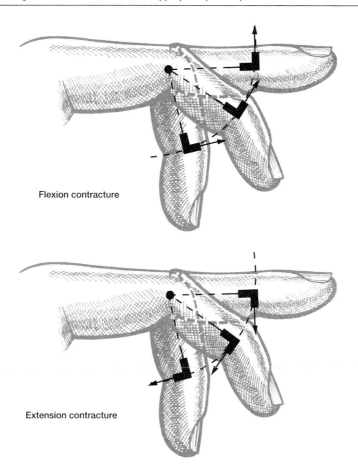

Flexion contracture

Extension contracture

Duration of Force Application

The mobility and flexibility of connective tissues that surround a joint may be affected by pathology associated with disease or trauma, by restricted mobility owing to injury to other regions of the limb or by prolonged immobilization. Connective tissue demonstrates elastic and viscous properties. Elastic properties allow recovery of shape and dimension after deformation. Viscous materials yield continuously under load and do not recover after unloading, commonly referred to as plastic deformation. When a force is

applied to connective tissue in order to gain greater motion, some of the elongation occurs in the elastic tissue elements and some in viscous elements. Thus, when stress is removed, the elastic deformation recovers whilst plastic deformation remains (Sapega et al., 1981). The stress must be applied for sufficient duration to produce synthesis of new tissue. Lengthening then becomes the result of tissue growth and not just deformation (Brand and Thompson, 1992).

The timing of force application, therefore, becomes a critical issue when mobilizing splints are used to correct deformity through the application of gentle forces. These forces cause tissue growth with an associated increase in passive range of motion. Some authors (Kottke *et al.*, 1966; Prosser, 1996) have investigated the association of duration and intensity of force application to resolution of joint contracture. Increased duration or prolonged moderate tension is significantly more effective in restoring passive motion than is intense stretching of short duration. High-stress, short-duration loading has a significantly higher risk of exceeding pain limits or producing evidence of tissue tearing. The study by Prosser (1996) found the single most significant factor in modifying shortened tissue was duration of force application.

CLINICAL APPLICATION

1. Maximize total end range time Maximizing total end range time (TERT) is the critical principle for lengthening of tissues and resolution of contracture. The hours per day that are available to apply the force to the relevant tissues should be identified. The 'dose' of treatment is the summation of all the time the joint is held at end range. It is determined by tolerance of the patient and the requirement for function or other treatment of the hand. Little empirical evidence exists to provide guides as to the most appropriate duration of splinting in terms of hours per day, and days per year in order to resolve tissue contracture.

2. Apply appropriate stress to modify tissues Dynamic splints apply two types of stress — compression at the site of force application and tension at the site of contracted tissues. The dose of stress must be sufficient to cause a therapeutic effect on the tissues under tension.

However, an excessive dose may produce complications, such as pain and inflammation not only in the tissues under tension but also in the compressed tissues at the site of force application. Little empirical evidence exists to provide guides as to the most appropriate torques or stress to apply in order to resolve tissue contracture.

3. Manipulate torque — modify distance of force application from axis Force applied at a greater distance from the joint axis will produce greater torque on the target tissues. Clinical judgement must be used to determine whether it is appropriate to increase or decrease torque.

4. Produce maximal torque from applied force — ensure perpendicular application Force applied at 90° to the long axis of the bone distal to the joint to be mobilized will be completely converted to rotational force and will avoid loss of effect to translational forces (Figure 13a).

Utilization of Mechanical Characteristics of Materials

Contour

Thermoplastic materials are thin and, when they are in flat sheets, they have little ability to resist bending. By curving and contouring the surface, the mechanical characteristics of the material are changed and it has greater strength to resist externally applied forces. A thin piece of metal may be easily bent if it is levered over a hard object but, if the same piece of metal was turned into a pipe, it is very difficult to bend. In the clinical situation, where the material must resist forces

Figure 13   Direction of application of actuating, manipulatory and stabilizing forces. (a) Perpendicular application of actuating force maximizes torque. (b) If forces are only applied at the sling and the dorsal component indicated by arrows in (a), rotation will occur around an undesired axis (the distal end of the dorsal restrict). Pressure will increase in magnitude towards the proximal edge of the sling and the distal edge of the dorsal restrict, and shear stress will occur in the finger at those points. The same situation will result when the sling does not pull at 90°, or when there is mechanical resistance at the PIP joint. (c) A reactive (stabilizing) force is required (volar splint component) to prevent unwanted movement and direct the applied actuating force to the target tissues. Pressure is now evenly distributed along the splint components.

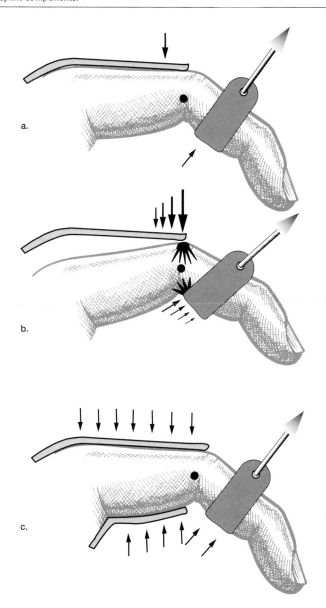

applied by the limb to maintain a prescribed position, and where enlarging the splint for strength is contraindicated for anatomical or functional reasons, contour is used to provide the necessary strength.

Friction

Friction is the force tending to prevent one body or object sliding on another. When a force is applied to an object which attempts to move the object, the force of friction prevents the object from moving (referred to as 'limiting friction'). If the force attempting to cause movement is strong enough, it overcomes the limiting friction and the object moves. Friction continues to operate to oppose the moving force and the objects exert an equal and opposite force on one another (referred to as 'normal reaction'). They do not slide freely, they 'rub'. Friction may be beneficial where it prevents unwanted movement or creates traction to enable work. It may be detrimental when it diminishes the efficiency of a machine or when one surface abrades another. In splinting, there are instances when it is better to increase friction and other times when the aim is to diminish friction. In both instances, it is usually a fine balance between the two to achieve beneficial results.

No surface is completely smooth but has depressions and projections. It is the interlocking of these tiny projections in the surfaces in contact that causes friction. Friction is consequently dependent on the type of surface, the size of surface area in contact and the normal reaction between the objects (the force holding the two together).

Friction between the splint and the limb is useful to prevent the splint from migrating, and is achieved by increasing the contact surface area (fit and contour) and increasing the normal reaction (e.g by applying straps). When forces that attempt to move the splint (as may occur when grasping) cannot overcome the friction, the splint and skin will move as one and the subcutaneous tissues will be exposed to sheer stress. If there is potential movement, it is better to provide an interface between the splint and the limb so the movement occurs between the splint and the interface. Similarly friction caused by movement of the splint on the limb will cause irritation to the skin. An interface layer between the two surfaces can assist in this regard. A removable hand sock will address this need. (This is the same principle as wearing socks with shoes.)

Low-profile outriggers are reported to require up to 40% more strength from the patient than do high profile outriggers to initiate and maintain active motion opposite to the dynamic assist direction of pull (Gyovai and Wright Howell, 1992). There is a similar loss in the amount of force that is generated by the dynamic force component which is transmitted to the target tissues. This is directly attributable to frictional drag at the traction system and outrigger pulley interface (Gyovai and Wright Howell, 1992; Boozer *et al.*, 1994). Loss of force secondary to friction between dynamic components of a splint and the outrigger or pulley plays a major role in influencing the amount of distal force applied (Gyovai and Wright Howell, 1992). Numerous attempts have been made to improve the drag and minimize friction from the traction–pulley interface. It is desirable to use a free and frictionless bar on the outrigger (Bell-Krotoski *et al.*, 1995). However, cost is a consideration in use of accessories such as wheel pulleys.

Mechanical Resistance

Resistance is often in the form of oedema or adhesions. In injuries where joint alignment is compromised, periarticular structures produce resistance to normal glide. Where there is mechanical resistance to an actuating force attempting to mobilize joints, the force will act on the point of least resistance. The force will cause rotation around an inappropriate axis (Figure 13b) unless additional applications of force direct the actuating force to the desired joints and restrict mobilization of inappropriate joints (Figure 13c).

Material Fatigue

In creating mechanical advantage in splints by increasing the length of the force arm (refer to Figures 6 and 7), there is a corresponding increase in the length of the moment arm around 'x' and therefore less force is required to produce a given amount of torque. Splints with longer proximal components are more prone to bending and, therefore, to material fatigue and fracture at the point adjoining the joint axis than are those with short proximal components. As mechanical advantage must not be compromised, the splint must be strong enough to withstand this rotational force. In the case of wrist splints, this point is also the narrowest part of the splint. Contour, including rolling edges, adds the required strength. Reinforcement may be necessary in some materials with low inherent strength.

Outrigger Profile

In splints designed with high-profile outriggers, the elastic traction component is attached directly to the outrigger. The height of the out-rigger is thus determined by the length of the elastic traction required. In low-profile splints, the outrigger acts as a pulley to redirect the line of pull, locating the elastic traction along the length of the splint (refer to Chapter 3 for further details). The pulley is a high point of friction.

High-profile outriggers require fewer adjustments to maintain 90° angle of pull than do low-profile outriggers when splints are applied to correct a joint contracture (Fess and Philips, 1987; Boozer et al., 1994). Complacency should be avoided when using high-profile outriggers. Any change of joint position will mean a loss of perpendicular pull.

Splinting used following metacarpophalangeal (MCP) joint replacement surgery requires a different thinking process in design. The objective is to maintain the MCP joints in extension and radial deviation, whilst still encouraging motion of the joints into flexion. This is one of the occasions where patients are encouraged to move in the direction opposite to the dynamic traction. As the MCP flexes, there is a loss of perpendicular line of pull of the traction force, which is translated to a compression force. Consequently, a low-profile splint provides greater stability to joints as they move opposite to the traction. This is advantageous in this case because of the inherent instability of the prostheses and the surgical repair.

Dynamic Component Characteristics

Two different types of splints use elastic bands and springs to provide a force to 'move' joints. Most common are splints that exert a constant tension on a restraining structure to mobilize shortened tissues and gain greater range of motion. The other type of splints use the force to position tissues whilst still allowing resisted movement in the direction opposite the traction, for example, Kleinert traction used following tendon repairs (Kleinert, *et al.*, 1975) and post-MCP arthroplasty splints.

The dynamic, or force, component of splints can be elastic bands or thread, mercery thread (elastic thread with a woven polyester coating that limits over stretching) or springs. These components have two variables, length and tension. Quality and thickness of the material determines its potential to generate tension, while length determines the potential elongation and distance through which tension can be generated. Chapter 3 describes the method of choice and application of the dynamic component.

Some dynamic components of splints are prone to fatigue or failure owing to their composition and the manner in which they are used:

1. Hysteresis is the loss of energy that occurs in an elastic material from repeated loading and unloading. In a material of poor quality or where the forces exceed the elastic capacity of the material, repeated loading results in a loss of ability to provide a controlled, repeatable force at a specified length, regardless of whether it is stretching or rebounding.

2. Length change from a sustained force may also occur when material quality is poor or the force exceeds the elastic capacity of the material. This is referred to as creep or deformation under constant load. Creep indicates the reliability of determining the force exerted at a given length after a given amount of time. Elastic bands are prone to creep and, therefore, require frequent adjustment to achieve a consistent force.

When structural fatigue occurs, there is a detect-able decrease in the tensile load throughout the load period. Length–tension relationships of materials become inconsistent and are unreliable when determining gradation of force.

Summary

The design of successful splints is dependent on a sound understanding of biomechanical principles. Pressure minimization, advantageous application of forces and beneficial use of material characteristics are the critical principles to be utilized.

References

Bell-Krotoski, JA, Breger-Lee, DE, Beach, RB (1995) Biomechanics and evaluation of the hand. In: Hunter, J, Makin, E, Callahan A. (eds) *Rehabilitation of the Hand*, 4th edn, pp. 153–184. St Louis: CV Mosby.

Boozer, JA, Sanson, MS, Soutas-Little, RW, *et al.* (1994) Comparison of the biomechanical motions and force involved in high-profile versus low-profile dynamic splinting. *Journal of Hand Therapy* 7: 171–182.

Brand, PW (1995) Mechanical factors in joint stiffness. *Journal of Hand Therapy* 8: 91–96.

Brand, PW, Hollister, A (1992) *Clinical Mechanics of the Hand*, 2nd edn. St Louis: Mosby — Year Book Inc.

Brand, PW, Thompson, DE (1992) Mechanical resistance. In: Brand, PW, Hollister, A (eds) *Clinical Mechanics of the Hand*, 2nd edn, pp. 92–128. St Louis: Mosby — Year Book Inc.

Fess, EE (1995) Splints: mechanics versus convention. *Journal of Hand Therapy* 8: 124–130.

Fess, EE, Philips, CA (1987) *Hand Splinting: Principles and Methods*, 2nd edn. St Louis: CV Mosby.

Gyovai, JE, Wright Howell, J (1992) Validation of spring forces applied in dynamic outrigger splinting. *Journal of Hand Therapy* 5: 8–15.

Kleinert, HE, Kutz, JE, Cohen, MJ (1975) Primary repair of zone 2 flexor tendon lacerations. In: *AAOS: Symposium on Tendon Surgery in the Hand*. St Louis: CV Mosby.

Kottke, FJ, Pauley, DL, Ptak, RA (1966) The rationale for prolonged stretching for correction of shortening of connective tissue. *Archives of Physical Medicine and Rehabilitation* 47: 345–352.

Prosser, R (1996) Splinting in the management of proximal interphalangeal joint flexion contracture. *Journal of Hand Therapy* 9: 378–386.

Sapega, AA, Quedenfeld, TC, Moyer, RA, *et al.* (1981) Biophysical factors in range of motion exercise. *The Physician and Sports Medicine* 9: 57–65.

Thompson, DE (1995) Dynamic properties of soft tissues and their interface with materials. *Journal of Hand Therapy* 8: 85–90.

3

Resources, Materials and Methods

Introduction
•
Resources
•
Materials
•
Methods
•
Conclusion

Introduction

Design and fabrication of splints requires a high degree of technical and practical competency. This chapter provides the information necessary to put into practice the skills to build and maintain a competency base. The information presented covers practical issues related to the physical environment, and to the materials and equipment used in a fabrication of hand splints.

Resources

Working Environment

In designing an effective working environment (either a new clinic or reorganization of an existing one), ergonomics, safety and efficiency must be considered.

OCCUPATIONAL HEALTH AND SAFETY

1. Hazards There are a number of safety hazards in the splinting environment. Close proximity of water and electricity, toxicity of plastics when heated, heat sources and sharp tools pose risks for the therapist and patient. Additionally, the repetitive and physically stressful nature of splinting predisposes the therapist's upper limbs and spine to misuse and overuse injuries. Good working habits, adequate worker fitness, and training and diligent application of occupational health procedures are essential to maintain a healthy working environment.

2. Ergonomic design The available work area must be designed to allow easy but safe movement from equipment to patient. Very few therapists have the luxury of designing the ideal area, thus design concepts and principles must be successfully incorporated into the available area. The three critical areas of patient, heat source and work area are best organized into a triangular configuration. Secondary areas can be arranged around this plan. Equipment, tools and materials must be positioned to provide easy access and speed of use. All work surfaces should be at ergonomically recommended heights (900 mm for standing, approximately 700 mm for sitting). The width of workbenches should be 450–600 mm, with frequently used tools positioned above the workbench ideally placed between 900 mm and 1500 mm (1800 mm maximum).

The position of the patient and the therapist for splint application must be considered to maximize comfort and effectiveness (Figure 1). The most common position for application is with the patient's elbow supported on a surface with the elbow flexed and the hand elevated (forearm mid-prone). Irrespective of the patient's and therapist's position, it is critical that the therapist is at the correct height to work safely on the patient's limb and is able to easily move around the limb (e.g. by mobile stool) to view and work on all aspects of the splint.

3. Hygiene There exists a high risk of cross-infection in hand practices. Tea tree oil has an

Figure 1 Ergonomic therapist – patient position. The therapist on the left is easily able to examine and treat the patient's upper limb. She is also in an ideal position to communicate with and respond to the patient.

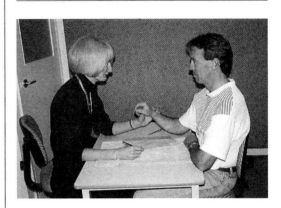

antibacterial action and is able to be used in the heating pan without altering any properties of thermoplastic material. Water should be changed daily or, in the case of splinting patients with acute wounds, before and after treatment. Heating pan and tools must be disinfected at least weekly. Standard infection control procedures should be adhered to: hand washing before and after treatment, using gloves in the presence of wounds, etc.

AESTHETIC CONSIDERATIONS

Consideration must also be given to the aesthetics of the environment. Therapists are treating patients who are often in pain, fearful or with chronic conditions. A pleasant, calm environment, without compromise to impressions of professional quality, will assist in putting patients at ease.

ENVIRONMENTAL ISSUES

Therapists should consider environmental factors in the choice of splinting materials. Some products are biodegradable and/or recyclable (e.g. Orfit®).

Fiscal Considerations

A successful practice requires effective accounting systems and methods. An efficient method of inventory and stock replenishment should be used.

Factoring the true cost of a splint, whether it be custom made or prefabricated, should include the time and expertise of the therapist, cost of materials, practice overheads, and depreciation on equipment and plant. Numerous attempts to achieve acceptable fabrication of a splint is very expensive in terms of the therapist's time, particularly if the result is unsuccessful. A prefabricated splint may appear to be expensive, but it requires less therapist time to prescribe and fit. However, there is cost involved in carrying stock or alternatively supplying on demand.

The true cost of a splint can only be measured once it successfully achieves the objectives for which it was designed. Financial outlay in material terms only, disregards the cost of labour time to manufacture, repair or replace the splint, for both the patient (such as lost work time to attend therapy) and therapist. Additionally, the patient may incur 'expense' in terms of suffering physical and psychological costs in a splint which fails to achieve its objectives or (in extreme cases) inflicts damage.

Equipment

The major items of equipment are heating sources, both wet and dry, to render low-temperature thermoplastic materials malleable. Hot water in a quantity sufficient to heat the majority of splint patterns must be regulated to the temperature appropriate to the materials being used. Large and deep electric frypans are adequate for most forearm/hand splints; purpose-designed hydrocollators and Suspans provide larger quantities of hot water.

There are a variety of heat guns available for hot air. Free-standing table models or hand-held models can be used for heating patterns, for spot heating for remoulding and to heat Velcro® adhesive and material surface for strap application. Funnel attachments are available to reduce the size of the hot air stream.

Tools

Good tools suited to the therapist's requirements increase the efficiency of splint fabrication. Tools must be well maintained, including regular sharpening to decrease the physical stress to the therapist's muscles and joints. Tools dedicated to splinting are advised to prevent frustrating losses effecting productivity, to prevent contamination with unacceptable substances and to ensure maintenance of good condition. Table 1 lists essential tools and their uses.

Materials

Thermoplastics

Thermoplastics are plastic and plastic-like materials that are affected by heat. Low-temperature thermoplastics, which soften at 60–70°C (140–160°F) are generally used to fabricate hand splints. An understanding of the properties of various materials is required for selection of the most appropriate material for a particular splint for a client. It allows the therapist to work with and take advantage of these properties for easy, accurate splint fabrication. In the same way that different types of clothes are made from different types of fabric, so it is with splints. The specific

Table 1
Tools

Tool	Use	Advantage	Recommended types
Shears	Cut patterns from large sheets of cold material	Fast, reduces waste, strong not precise	Heavy duty shears, tin snips
Scissors	Cutting materials	Accurate, allows specialized finishing techniques, proficient use requires practice	Blunt-nose surgical, large-handle Fisker, curved Mayo
Hole punch	Punching holes – Velcro®, rivets, dynamic pulleys, thumb/finger holes	Neat, fast, even, smooth edge	Revolving leather punch
Riveter	Securing two-part rivets	Less expensive than adhesive Velcro®, still required for some attachments	Hand press or bench mounted
Small vice	Bending outriggers	Safer, stronger, faster, more precise, less stressful than by hand	Bench press or small vice
Pliers	Bending, cutting outriggers	Safer, stronger, faster, more precise, less stressful than by hand	Square nose, round nose
Stanley trimmer	Cutting straight lines	Easier, less stress than scissors	
Awl	Marking splinting material	Aesthetically preferable to pen	
Beveler	Smoothing edges	Useful on thick splinting materials	
Jigs	Making wire springs, outriggers	Safer, stronger, faster, more precise, less stressful than by hand	See Figure 2

properties of each material lend themselves to the most appropriate design and construction techniques.

There is a wide variety of splinting materials on the market. Currently, it is appropriate to consider splinting materials as having plastic-, rubber-, or plastic- and rubber-like properties (Breger-Lee and Buford, 1992; Breger-Lee, 1995). General features and their advantages and disadvantages are reviewed. Table 2, which is intended only as a guide, identifies the properties of various materials. As development of new products is ongoing, therapists must diligently update their knowledge.

Features of Thermoplastics

GENERAL CHARACTERISTICS

Each material has different properties when cold and when heated. The features when cold give some indication of the properties of the splint once fabricated, and include thickness, rigidity

Table 2
Thermoplastic Splinting Materials
There is such a wide range of low-temperature thermoplastics available that it is impossible and confusing to describe them all. However, if the material base is known, the characteristics of a particular material can be predicted (Breger-Lee and Buford, 1992). Materials are available in different grades, sizes and thickness, with or without perforations, different sizes and density of perforations, in different colours, with different activation temperatures and with special features. It is vital to read the manufacturer's instructions prior to using materials to achieve the best performance from the material.

Base	Examples	Characteristics
Transpolyisoprene (TPI)	Orthoplast Ezeform Synergy Leodisplint Multiform isoprene NCM Spectrum	• Rubber based or rubber-like • Requires more force to mould • Low conformability • Not influenced by gravity • No elastic memory but poor stretch means original shape can be approximated on reheating • Retain heat for longer than plastic based materials • Do not become more pliable with overheating – lose rubber properties • Adhere when hot, not when cooled • Require bonding agents for adherence
Polycaprolactone (PCL)	Polyform NCM Clinic Orthoplast II Multiform plastic	• Plastic based or plastic-like • Highly mouldable and drapable • Overheating destroys properties • Gravity overstretches overheated material • Short heating time • Self-adherent or surface coated • Surface coated require bonding agent
TPI/PCL blended	Polyflex/ Sansplint XR NCM Preferred	• Plastic/rubber combinations • Conformability is between TPI and PCL • Characteristics depend on blend • Treat as if plastic based
Materials that turn clear	Aquaplast Multiform clear Orfit	• Treat as if plastic based • Self-adherent • Elastic memory • Orfit has lowest activation temperature
Other thermoplastics	Hexcelite Sanlite	• Have the handling characteristics of plastic-based materials but no stretch • Lightweight open-weave material which is fabricated with a spun-fibre lining • Adherent

and the presence of perforations. This has implications for the patient and how they will use the splint.

The properties of the material when heated suggest how that material will respond during the fabrication process. This has relevance to splint design and what the material is suitable for, the fabrication techniques that can be used and the unique needs of the client (e.g. the aged, children, or the presence of wounds).

ACTIVATION TEMPERATURE

The temperature at which thermoplastic splinting materials become pliable is referred to as the activation temperature. It is important to note this temperature and set the thermostat of the heating pan accordingly, as the properties of some materials may change if overheated.

Materials may lose properties such as the ability to reach true pliability when heated, lose stretchability (e.g. Orfit®), become overstretched (e.g. Sansplint XR®/Polyflex®) or lose rigidity when cold. Colour changes may occur in some materials. Materials which are transparent when heated may lose this characteristic and remain opaque. These problems may also occur with some materials if they are reheated several times.

With a lower activation temperature, there is a lower risk of burns to both the therapist and patient. This is an important consideration for those patients with fragile skin, particularly children, the elderly, and post-trauma in the presence of grafts and burns. It also decreases the working time for moulding as the material cools and hardens in a few minutes.

MOULDABILITY AND DRAPABILITY

Once heated, materials exhibit varying degrees of rigidity and mouldability (drapability). Highly drapable materials (e.g. Sansplint XR®/Polyflex®) are recommended in acute phase post-injury or in the presence of significant pain when the patient's tissues can not tolerate any force being applied during fabrication. Highly drapable materials require gravity to assist moulding with little effort from the therapist to achieve a precise mould to the contours of the limb. However, this material is difficult to use without the assistance of gravity as bandaging is not recommended. Caution is required when handling this type of material as

it can be easily stretched and the surface of the material marks very easily. More rigid materials require constant pressure to achieve good conformity and generally require bandaging to the limb.

ELASTIC MEMORY

A material which has the ability to return to its original size and shape when reheated has elastic memory. Thus splints can be completely remoulded to accommodate changes due to reduction of oedema or changes in range of motion as in the case of serial splinting. It also has benefits for the novice as mistakes are easily rectified by reworking the same piece of material. Also remoulding is possible, saving expense in material outlay when repeated splint application is required over time.

When using material with elastic memory, partial melting can result in significant changes in contour and shape which can distort the original design. It is better to become proficient at achieving all desired characteristics in one mould, something that can only be achieved by practice.

COATING AND SELF-ADHERENCE

Many of the materials have a coating on the surface which prohibits self-adherence when activated. This lessens the risk of the splint material adhering to itself, the patient or dressings when activated during moulding. Cut edges will still adhere. Coatings have to be removed either with solvents or sandpaper prior to attempting to adhere another splint component such as outrigger bonds or straps.

Materials without a coating are referred to as self-adherent. They simplify splint fabrication through eliminating the need for bandaging as they adhere to the patient or to themselves when used circumferentially. Straps and other components adhere without requiring solvents or bonding agents.

Self-adherent materials must remain wet while moulding to prevent the material from adhering to itself and other products. Gauze or stockinette can be used over post-operative dressings so the thermoplastic adheres to it and not the dressing.

TRANSPARENCY WHEN HEATED

Some materials become transparent when heated, which is often claimed to be advantageous as anatomical landmarks and skin blanching can be seen whilst moulding; however, the benefit in reality is negligible. Transparency allows the therapist to determine easily when the material is activated, saving time and avoiding the risk of overheating.

PERFORATIONS

Transpiration of water via the skin is an ongoing process. Therefore, the application of splinting material which prevents the normal evaporative process may lead to accumulation of moisture with maceration of the skin. Splinting materials with perforations may be cooler, drier and more comfortable. The splinting materials allow the skin to breathe only in those locations with holes. If splints are to be effective in reducing the temperature and allowing evaporation, the holes need to be sufficiently large and spaced at close intervals.

One disadvantage of maxi-perforated splinting materials is that skin may be pushed through the perforations and cause shear at the edges. Perforated materials should not be stretched during fabrication, otherwise the holes may be enlarged and strength properties lost. Perforated materials have been shown to break down in areas

of high stress (Breger-Lee and Buford, 1992). The edges of perforated materials must be smoothed as cutting causes uneven and sharp edges to be formed.

Neoprene

Commonly referred to as wetsuit material, this material comprises an internal rubber layer of various thickness and external nylon layers in a range of colours. It is cut and sewn to fabricate splints. The material does not limit motion and is bulky, hot and not well tolerated in warm climates.

Contour is achieved by the pattern design and rigidity gained by additional reinforcement from thermoplastic inserts. This material is commonly used for splints for very young children where the bulk of the material offers enough restriction to position joints, as a means to maintain warmth surrounding a joint (e.g. post-fracture), and for persons with arthritis because of the gentle support and warmth.

Leather

Three-millimetre-thick stiff, natural leather is used for work-based splints to immobilize the wrist in environments where thermoplastic materials can not be used (in the presence of heat and petroleum-based chemicals). The basis of patterns is similar to that for neoprene. Wet leather is moulded directly to the limb and bandaged, then allowed to dry for approximately 24 hours. Straps are riveted or glued. The leather can be sealed and polished.

Plaster of Paris

Plaster is a cost-effective, easy method of fabricating circumferential serial splints, especially for the elbow and proximal interphalangeal (PIP) joint. It allows tissue to breath so it does not macerate the skin and it can be used over lacerations and ulcers. Finger plasters are applied without underlying protection. Larger plasters require cast padding. The plaster is rolled on without any compression until the required thickness is achieved and then smoothed off with moistened hands giving particular attention to the edges. Small splints can be soaked off, larger splints require bivalving with a plaster saw.

Plaster, in bandage form, is gauze impregnated with plaster (calcium sulphate). Plaster setting involves an exothermic chemical reaction, which results in the hydration of calcium sulphate to produce gypsum. The rate of this reaction is largely dependent upon the amount of water incorporated in the dry plaster and the temperature of this water. For application, the plaster should be saturated with water but not 'dripping' wet. Excessively dry or wet plaster yields poor crystallization. Ideally, the dipping temperature should be between 25° and 30°C (77–86°F). Curing time is dependent on temperature, humidity and, most importantly, adequate air circulation around the cast. Strength (gypsum crystal interlocking) depends upon the speed of setting, the water content and the amount of motion during cure. During setting, water is incorporated into the gypsum crystals resulting in cast expansion. This expansion enhances intimate moulding to anatomical contours. Excess water gradually evaporates and most is lost within 4 hours. Thus, for best casting results:

1. Use water between 25° and 30°C (77–86°F).
2. Apply material smoothly with the minimum number of layers possible.
3. Prevent motion during setting.
4. Do not insulate from free access to air by placing a towel or bandage over a freshly applied plaster.

Lycra®

Lycra® has long been used in the manufacture of pressure garments for oedema control and scar management. Incorporation of various Lycra® fabrics into soft wrist splinting has been reported in the literature. Recent developments in the use of Lycra® in dynamic splints to address neuromuscular problems associated with hyper- and hypotonicity offer splinting options by providing stability whilst allowing mobility.

Lycra® offers the potential to manufacture splints with a range of mobility and rigidity. Where multiple joints are involved, hard splinting would prevent movement to the point of loss of hand function, whereas a Lycra® splint can be fabricated to allow the appropriate movement in prescribed joints. The elastic nature of Lycra® can offer enough support for unstable joints in rheumatoid arthritis when total restriction is contraindicated or functionally unacceptable.

Lycra® is available in a range of strengths, weights and colours. It breathes but can become hot to wear. To make a garment, a pattern is required and the pieces are overlocked together. Numerous brands of prefabricated Lycra®-based splints are available.

Strapping Materials

Straps are required to provide stability and to secure the splint to the body in the prescribed position. Distal movement of the splint, especially rotation, will compromise the desired outcome and can be controlled with appropriate choice and application of strapping to distribute forces correctly. Velcro® is perhaps the most common form of strapping material but other options are available.

VELCRO®

Velcro® is available in various widths, with or without elasticity, in various colours and with or without adhesive backing. Although both hook and pile Velcro® is available with adhesive backing, only adhesive hook Velcro® is generally required for splints. Choice of colour should reflect consideration of aesthetics and the patient's preferences. Choice of width reflects functional considerations.

Velcro® is a brand name and is a good quality product. Cheaper products with similar properties are available; however, durability and performance is directly related to cost.

BETAPILE™

When skin is fragile, Betapile™ may be used in conjunction with hook Velcro®. It is available in various widths and consists of brown brushed nylon bonded to two sides of 5 mm-thick foam. Betapile™ has slight stretch and, therefore, can not be used where a firm strap is required.

COTTON OR DACRON WEBBING WITH VELCRO® TABS

These materials are tough, durable and non-elastic. Hook and pile Velcro® and buckles must be sewn on. The straps can only be attached to the splint with rivets. Webbing is advised when straps must be long-lasting and strong.

Principles of Strapping Design and Application

Consideration of strap application must be included throughout the design process to ensure a professional, aesthetically pleasing and functionally acceptable product. The position of application should be carefully determined prior to actual application, for once most straps are attached, they are difficult to remove and inappropriate positioning may render the splint ineffective.

BIOMECHANICAL CONSIDERATIONS

Adherence to biomechanical principles of splint design, as described in Chapter 2, is essential. Critical issues pertaining to strap application are:

1. Straps apply at least one critical component of the force couple exerted by the splint to maintain the correct position. Thus strap width must be generous.
2. The angle of application must allow for the tapering shape of the forearm (see Figure 3 in Chapter 2). Thus straps sit flush with the skin providing firm, equal pressure distribution avoiding shear stress.
3. Straps are unable to contour to concave or convex surfaces. Bony prominences are convex in more than one plane, therefore, uneven pressure results when straps are applied. Elastic Velcro® does not solve this problem.
4. The position of application of straps should maximize the mechanical advantage offered by the splint. A splint that requires a proximal component to be two-thirds the length of the forearm should not be compromised by a proximal strap positioned only halfway along the length.

ANATOMICAL CONSIDERATIONS

1. Apply straps acknowledging that the architecture of the hand does change with motion. Movement should not be impaired by strap width or location.
2. Protection of circulatory integrity. Straps are liable to impair lymphatic and venous drainage,

or compromise arterial status unless width allows adequate distribution of pressure and placement does not jeopardize critical structures.

3. Protect skin integrity. Consider fragility of the skin and tolerance to wear when choosing strap material, placement and width. Permeable materials allow water and air exchange, and thus lessen the risk of maceration. However, they are harder to keep clean and pose an infection risk (the thermoplastic is not permeable and can be disinfected).

FUNCTIONAL CONSIDERATIONS

1. Prescription of amount of Velcro® This should be prescribed in accordance with the requirements of the patient and the therapist's objectives. Too much Velcro® may prove difficult to undo for those patients with diminished hand function. Small amounts are acceptably strong and secure. Make the hook Velcro® a little thinner and smaller than the associated pile Velcro® as this will result in the hook being completely covered by the pile, particularly for those patients with diminished manipulation skills. Full coverage of hook Velcro® is essential, as exposure may result in skin irritation or trauma, or snagging against other materials.

2. Ease of application and removal Consideration must be given to the patient's bilateral upper limb function when determining the orientation of straps for the direction of fastening and unfastening to enable the patient to apply the splint independently. Patients with diminished hand function may need to sweep the opposite wrist or forearm around the splint to fasten or unfasten straps, or even need to use their teeth. The ends of the pile Velcro® must be slightly longer than the underlying hook to afford full coverage and give adequate grip to unfasten. Those with bilateral injuries or diminished manipulation skills require strap adaptations or modified prehension patterns to simplify the task of fastening and unfastening. Alternatively, there may be occasions when straps are applied to make splint removal more difficult as in the case of young children.

3. Comfort and function In firmly securing the splint to the hand, comfort should not be overlooked as this will significantly affect compliance. The hook Velcro® should be applied on to the thermoplastic, facing away from the patient's skin, with the pile Velcro® applied at the edges of the thermoplastic facing towards the skin. This prevents discomfort, irritation or trauma to the patient's skin from the rough hook material.

4. Durability The straps should withstand the constant wear the splint will receive.

AESTHETIC CONSIDERATIONS

The strapping components should be of the same colour, and of a colour to match or complement the thermoplastic as closely as possible. The exception should be where contrasting colours are aesthetically acceptable to the patient. For example, white hook Velcro® on white thermoplastic with blue pile Velcro® to replicate the patient's football team colours. The ends of both the hook and the pile Velcro® should be cut to the desired length and curved for neatness.

Lining Materials

Lining should only be prescribed if it is essential. Linings are problematic as the soft nature leads to breakdown and shortens the life of the splint.

Many adhesive-backed lining materials are very difficult to apply and remove, so consider this fact prior to application. Table 3 presents commonly used linings and their properties.

INDICATIONS FOR USE OF LINING MATERIALS

Comfort Plastic materials are not comfortable to wear next to the skin, particularly if heat or perspiration is a problem. Skin maceration may result. Splints are often lined to minimize this problem but these linings quickly become soiled with perspiration and grime. If the lining becomes wet, it will remain so for extended periods, risking skin integrity. The lining is difficult to clean and, once wet, difficult to remove. Replacement is expensive, time consuming and often difficult. To increase the comfort of shoes, we wear socks or stockings – consider a similar application of cotton stockinette for the hand. A length of nylon stocking, or thin cotton socks overlocked at either end may be equally comfortable.

Linings are either closed cell or open cell in structure. Liquids, perspiration, odours and bacteria do not penetrate the surface of closed cell materials but they do not breathe. They are, however, easier to clean. Open cell materials breathe but will absorb liquids and so are unhygienic. Also they easily stain and become odoriferous.

To enhance pressure distribution The addition of lining increases pressure as opposed to decreasing it, and should not be seen as a means of improving the fit of a poorly designed and fabricated splint. If lining is deemed necessary to improve pressure distribution, allowance should be made for it in initial fabrication. Some linings

are adhered to the thermoplastic prior to heating and moulding but they significantly affect the qualities of the thermoplastic. Linings that do not bottom out have the ability to absorb press and reduce shear stress (using a stockinette liner decreases shear as movement occurs between the splint and the liner rather than the skin). Any lining that bottoms on compression (squeeze foam between thumb and finger to test) is inappropriate to address pressure or shear. All linings minimize splint migration by increasing friction between the splint and skin but, therefore, require careful monitoring of the skin for shear problems. Splints should not be partially lined as this alters the skin/splint interface and causes areas of shear stress.

Maintenance of skin integrity Clients with sensitive skin may require the splint to be lined. Lining is a special consideration in splint fabrication for persons with an allergy to splinting material, with fragile skin, such as in rheumatoid arthritis or following a skin graft, or with sensory loss who can not feel skin irritation.

Contact Media

Where pressure needs to be applied to skin to modify a scar, a splint is unable to conform to the scar surface to give even pressure distribution. Likewise, linings have inadequate conformability and may be contraindicated for some scars. Contact media, such as silastic elastomer or Ottoform, may be utilized under the splint, creating true congruity and offering a beneficial side effect in softening the scar. These media can also be used for precise positioning of joints of the hand within the splint, in cases of rheumatoid arthritis and severe trauma.

Table 3
Lining Materials

Material	Description/uses	Application	Thickness and size	Colour	Durability	Stretch and contour	Ease of removal	Surface texture	Cell structure	Compressibility	Special features
Adhesive fleecy web	Fabric-surfaced lining	Post-moulding	22.5 × 45 × 0.2 cm	Pink	Low	Moderate to high	Easy	Soft, fluffy	Open	Thin, bottoms out	
Adhesive moleskin	Fabric-surfaced lining	Post-moulding	30 cm × 5 m roll	Flesh	High	Low	Medium	Finer than fleecy web	Open	The thinnest lining, bottoms out	Recommended for allergy to thermoplastics
Adhesive polycushion	Soft-foam padding	Pre- or post-moulding	3 mm, 6 mm thick	Beige	Moderate	Low	Very difficult	Soft foam	Closed – will not absorb perspiration	Resists bottoming out	Washable Available in low tack for easier removal
Adhesive cushion-flex	Serial splint	Pre- or post-moulding	3 mm thick	White	High	Very low	Difficult	Firm, smooth	Closed – will not absorb perspiration	Resists bottoming out	Washable

Hexalon Synthetic cast padding Sofban	To line porous material such as hexalite Under plaster casts	Pre-moulding – heat material and lining together then cut pattern	Negligible thickness	White	Low – pills up and wears in susceptible areas Tears easily	Very high	Can pull out most but never all of it Cannot reline	Soft, fluffy	Porous, spun dacron or cotton fibre Absorbs moisture	Bottoms out	Non-adhesive Bonds to materials that become tacky when heated Washable
Elastonett	Use under splint like a sock Cut hole for thumb	Separate and removable	Various circum-ferences – 5 cm for hand	White, biege	Will last numerous washes, if edges over-stitched	High	Take off hand and wash	Various according to brand	Open cell woven polycotton	No cushioning properties	Various brands, different firmness

Miscellaneous Hardware

HOOKS

Although there are many devices available from suppliers to tether and align dynamic traction, dress hooks and eyes are economical and convenient. They are available in a large range of sizes in haberdashery shops. Hooks can be heated and embedded in most thermoplastics (some require a small piece of thermoplastic bonded over the top) to attach the traction force component. The eye may need to be bent at 90° at the waist (for thinner materials) and then attached in the same way to create a pulley guide for the traction system.

OUTRIGGERS

Outriggers require ease of adjustment to ensure that the angle of pull of traction remains at 90°. Dynamic outriggers may be constructed from a range of materials.

1. Metal Brass welding rod (3.2 or 1.6 mm in diameter) or 1.6 mm-diameter stainless steel rod is cost effective, aesthetically acceptable, and easy to bend, cut and modify. Gauge 13 spring wire is used for spring coils. These metals are bent using vices, pliers and jigs (Figure 2). A narrow, small strip of thermoplastic should be attached to the larger outriggers into which holes can be punched as pulleys for low-profile traction systems. Metal eyes should be embedded into the inferior curve to reduce friction against the nylon thread.

2. Thermoplastic In order to achieve the desired strength, the design is extremely bulky and, therefore, unattractive and expensive.

Figure 2   Dynamic splint outriggers. Examples of outrigger styles for individual finger outriggers and for multiple finger outriggers, and the jigs used to create them. Pliers, jigs and vices should be used wherever possible to protect the tissues of the therapist's hands. The safety pin is useful as an individual finger outrigger for small finger splints.

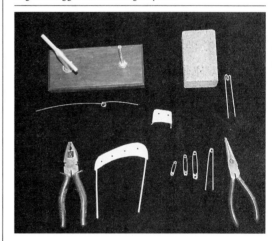

3. Orfitubes® The traction is completely encased within a tube. Expense is an issue with these tubes but aesthetically they are very acceptable. Orfitubes® are cold formable to the desired length of the splint. The maximum length of elastic traction can be used as no pulley is required.

DYNAMIC (FORCE) COMPONENTRY

The traction unit for a low-profile splint consists of the cuff, an inelastic component (usually nylon thread) and an elastic component (either elastic bands or elastic thread). The length of the cuff is sufficient to cradle the digit. The nylon thread is secured independently to each side of the cuff with sufficient length to allow the traction unit to glide through the pulley created by the outrigger. The elastic component has the following two variables.

1. Tension Quality and thickness of the material determines its potential to generate tension.

This tension is translated to force applied to tissues.

2. Length Length determines the potential elongation and distance through which tension can be generated. This distance is critical for allowing a full prescribed range of motion.

When dynamic traction is used in a splint, the therapist needs to know how much tension is generated when the component is stretched to a predetermined point. When the same amount of force is applied to components of differing thicknesses and lengths, different elongation results. Greater elongation occurs in longer elastic bands when compared to short bands. Similarly, thinner elastic bands elongate more than thick bands. If the components are stretched to a similar length, the tensions generated vary widely. This is clinically significant as it demonstrates that the component has an optimal range of lengths at which it can exert useful tension. Short bands produce larger tension with less excursion than do longer bands, which make short bands inappropriate in many applications.

Determination of length–tension of elastic traction A distinction must be made regarding the therapeutic rationale and outcome objectives for dynamic traction as this will modify the determination of force range. Where the objective is to address deficits in passive range of motion (PROM) and influence tissue length, the critical issue is total end range time (TERT). In these splints, the appropriate force is determined to be that which will maintain the joint at its end range and is of the correct magnitude to impact positively on tissue change (see Chapters 1 and 2). In this instance it defeats the objective to allow movement against the traction, therefore, the second measurement described below in

point 3 (antagonist force) is inappropriate. When the patient is required to move against the splint traction in a repetitive manner within the prescribed range of joint motion (e.g. to achieve the therapeutic objective of minimizing adhesion formation), the outlined procedure is appropriate.

1. As each dynamic component has a different length–tension curve, therapists must complete a quick once-off exercise (Figure 3) of plotting the curve for the range of components they use. When low-profile splinting is used, this exercise should be performed through a pulley system as the loss of force to friction must be acknowledged. These graphs are then used to determine the force generated at each point of elongation (see Figure 4).
2. Determine the range of excursion required. This is a linear measurement of the joint range of motion (Figure 5).
3. Determine the force range required. The minimum force is that which is required to maintain the joint in the prescribed position, measured

Figure 3 Plotting length–tension curves for dynamic components. Using a Haldex gauge (or other calibrated force gauge) and ruler, plot the forces produced at various points of elongation of the dynamic component. This quick exercise should be completed for every component the therapist commonly uses.

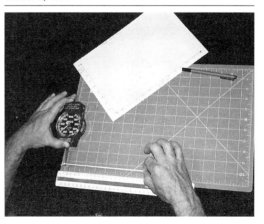

Figure 4 Length–tension curve of a 50 mm elastic band. This graph demonstrates the curvilinear relationship of length and tension force in a 50 mm elastic band. This curve is used to determine the correct application of dynamic traction to achieve the desired force application. For example, if the range of force required is 150–250 g, identify this on the vertical axis (indicated by a). Project these values across to the curve and then down to the horizontal axis (indicated by b). The range identified by b is 125–162 mm. Therefore, the excursion of the elastic band which will achieve the desired force range equals 125–162 mm. Traction must be applied with the band elongated to 125 mm. This component will allow 37 mm linear range of movement at the targeted joint.

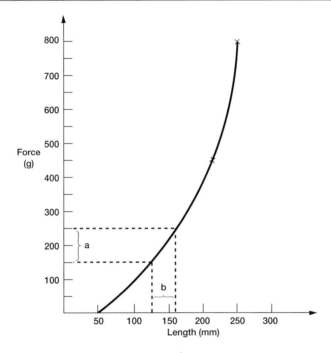

with a force gauge (Figure 6). The maximum force is that which the antagonist muscle group is able to generate in opposition to the prescribed position. A clinical decision may be required in the event of the antagonists being unable to oppose the minimum force. Modifications may be required to the therapeutic regime to address this issue. The maximum force should not exceed the safe limit for application of force to living tissues. The recommended upper limit is 300 g force.

4. Use the length–tension curves to determine the appropriate dynamic component to use and the point of elongation at which to apply the system (an example is demonstrated on Figure 4).

5. Determine the most suitable type of outrigger and its height. In high profile (vertical traction) the outrigger is the point of attachment of the dynamic component. In low-profile (horizontal traction) the outrigger is used as a pulley. The suspension sling is attached to nylon thread which runs through the pulley and then attaches to the dynamic component. This sits horizontal to the splint and is tethered proximally. The practice of applying horizontal traction to a high outrigger nullifies the design benefits of low-profile splint.

Consider the measurement determined at point 2, and the suspension/sling system. For example, if 40 mm excursion is required and the sling requires 10 mm clearance, a high-

Figure 5   Linear measurement of joint range of motion. The excursion that is required by the dynamic component to allow the desired range of joint motion is easily determined. x = joint axis; a = point of application of traction; b = distance x − a; c = joint range of motion; d = linear distance. Identify the desired joint range of motion (c) according to the prescribed end ranges the traction is to provide. To convert this angular length to a linear length, draw the simple diagram as indicated in the bubble with the appropriate measurements. Measure the linear length d, and add 20% to allow for increasing range and for the extra length in the curve. For example, if d = 30 mm, the range of excursion required = 36 mm. If the elastic band demonstrated in Figure 4 was used, it provides enough excursion for the desired joint range and force application, but with little room for error. If it did not provide adequate excursion, a different component must be selected.

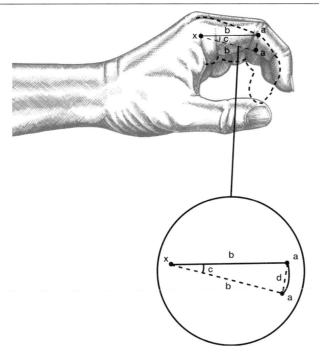

Figure 6   Force range requirements. Using a force gauge, measure the amount of force required to maintain the joint in the prescribed position. If the therapy objectives require joint motion, measure the force the patient can generate against the gauge to achieve this joint motion.

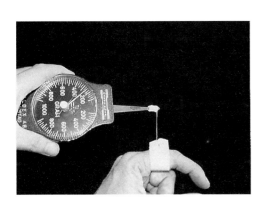

profile outrigger needs to sit 50 mm from the point of traction application. This is not a consideration in low-profile outriggers as the outrigger sits as close as possible without compromising motion and the sling system requires less space.

6. The design of splint must accommodate the desired excursion of the elastic traction and not vice versa. Low-profile splints require a longer base to accommodate the traction system but this is often mechanically advantageous anyway. The nylon thread needs only be long enough to yield full excursion through the pulley, allowing the longest possible dynamic component. This system permits flexibility in

the choice of dynamic component as it provides a greater range of safe length to desired tension.

FINGER CUFFS

Dynamic splint cuffs are used to apply force to the fingers to address passive motion deficits. Selection of material requires the same consideration as other splint components with regard to skin integrity. Cuffs must be durable, comfortable and resist stretching. Velcro®, suede or leather may be chosen. For strong functional loops (e.g. radial nerve palsy splint) leather is appropriate. Suede is softer and more compliant and is a better choice for patients with frail skin. Biomechanical principles must be adhered to, specifically pressure distribution and the avoidance of shear stress.

Constructing the Dynamic Component

PROCEDURE FOR A SINGLE DIGIT

1. Identify the dynamic component to be used in the traction system.
2. Design and fabricate the appropriate splint base to stabilize the body part and provide a base for attachment of the outrigger.
3. Apply selected straps to secure the splint but not to obstruct construction or placement of the outrigger.
4. Fabricate the outrigger.
   (a) Roughly measure the length of outrigger metal required (the minimum is double the length of the bones proximal and distal to the joint to be mobilized).
   (b) At the mid-point construct the pulley by either coiling with pliers or bending an 'M' shape with a jig (Figure 2).
   (c) Make a digit cuff and attach nylon thread.

(d) Secure the splint to the hand and place the cuff on the digit.
(e) Place the outrigger on the splint with the nylon thread through the pulley. Mobilize the joint to its end range using the tension on the cuff. Adjust the position of the outrigger to achieve a perpendicular pull by the traction system on the digit. Mark the location of the outrigger on the splint base. Trim the excess length off the outrigger and contour it to the splint base. Heat the outrigger over the heat gun and position it on splint base. Secure it with an additional piece of splinting material.
(f) Determine the maximum length of nylon thread required, then add the dynamic component to the traction.
(g) Heat a small dress hook and secure it to the splint base at the point predetermined by the length tension required by the traction.
(h) A pulley, to maintain traction alignment close to the splint base, can be made from the 'eye' of a dress hook and secured to the splint base.

PROCEDURE FOR MULTIPLE DIGITS

A single outrigger is used for several digits where the contributing pathology and the deficits in joint range of motion in each digit are similar. Where there is disparity in either of these factors, individual outriggers are made to address each digit.

1. Identify the dynamic component to be used in the traction system.
2. Design and fabricate the appropriate splint base to stabilize the body part and provide a base for attachment of the outrigger.
3. Apply selected straps to secure the splint but not to obstruct construction or placement of the outrigger.

4. Fabricate the outrigger.

(a) Roughly measure the length of the outrigger metal required (the minimum is the width of the digits involved plus twice the length of the hand and/or forearm splint base).

(b) Make digit loops and attach a length of nylon thread to each loop.

(c) Secure the splint to the hand and place a loop on the most radial digit involved.

(d) Bend the outrigger metal at approximately 90° at the distal radial corner allowing sufficient length for the radial arm of the outrigger to contour the splint base.

(e) Mobilize the most radial digit involved to its end range using the tension on the cuff. Determine the length of the outrigger from the splint base to the intersection of the traction to achieve a perpendicular pull on the digit. This location is marked. The outrigger metal rod is then shaped to contour the radial side of the splint base. The outrigger is then shaped to accommodate the width of the involved digits following the architecture of the hand. The ulnar arm of the outrigger is shaped similarly to that of the radial arm. Again location on the splint base is marked. The excess length of the outrigger is trimmed prior to securing it to the splint base with additional splinting material. The protective non-adhesive coating on some splinting materials must be removed prior to bonding the outrigger.

(f) A thin piece of thermoplastic material is then moulded over the distal end of the outrigger. The position can be varied through an arc of 180° to ensure the correct angle of pull on the traction. A hole is punched in this splinting material to create the pulley for each digit.

(g) The 'eyes' of dress hooks are heated over the heat gun and positioned in the thermoplastic around the holes to minimize friction and prevent the traction cutting through the splinting material.

(h) A small dress hook is melted into the thermoplastic at the proximal end of the splint.

(i) Attach the dynamic component to the nylon thread of each traction system. Thread the traction through the corresponding hole in the outrigger and secure to the hook.

Methods

Pattern Design

Pattern design is an integral part of prescription, requiring concurrent analysis of material choice, fabrication technique and essential componentry. Essentially the problem is similar to dressing making in that a three-dimensional splint is manufactured from a two-dimensional material.

There is a direct correlation between the precision of the pattern taken and the outcome of the splint. Taking a good pattern is the first stage of successful splinting. Specific patterns are discussed in the appropriate chapter. It is vital to read all the instructions with the diagrams and have an understanding of the procedure prior to commencing. Pattern making, similar to all aspects of splint fabrication, is a skill to be practised.

The patterns presented in the following chapters are detailed and complete to allow an inexperienced therapist to design a pattern with little prior experience. As clinical competency increases, the need to identify all points and dimensions of the hand may not be necessary.

METHODS OF PATTERN MAKING

The requirements for patterns vary with the material. The type of material used will govern the choices available in pattern making. The more rigid materials require more precise patterns.

In order to take a pattern you will need a piece of paper towel or plastic sheet (plastic is more resistant to tearing and is, therefore, more appropriate for use with children or non-compliant patients), pencils, pens, ruler, scissors and tape measure.

1. Landmark, pattern and apply This is the more precise design technique. Identify appropriate landmarks and shape the pattern using those landmarks. This pattern must be cut out from the paper or plastic, and applied to the limb to check the fit prior to transferring it to the splinting material. If the pattern is inaccurate or incorrect, it will have direct implications for the success of splint fabrication.

2. Rough pattern, stretch and mould The unique properties of highly malleable thermoplastic materials allows stretch and contour without loss of properties. A rough pattern only is required, and this is stretched and pulled into position. Excess material is trimmed after moulding. If these materials are stretched too far, they become thin and lose strength. They should be stretched slowly to prevent this occurring.

Fabrication Techniques

CREATING HOLES

In materials with a high degree of stretch and drape, creating openings for digits requires only a small hole punched with a leather punch. This is stretched, rolled or smoothed to the appropriate size (Figure 7). Soft, gentle and slow strokes are advised in materials without elastic memory to avoid over-stretching the hole and thinning the material.

CUTTING HOT SEAMS

Many splints, such as cylindrical splints and hand-based splints, can take advantage of properties that allow a neat seam to be created. Materials need to be highly drapable and stretchable, and be either self-adherent or adherent with pressure or on cutting. The material is pulled around the limb and the two edges adhered or held together where the seam is desired. Holding the scissor blades closely to the skin surface, cut with long, smooth strokes (Figure 8). The cut edges will bond together to form a flat neat seam. For the neatest results, care should be taken to ensure the material is pulled together and cut in a straight line, usually aligning with some limb axis. The seam may need reinforcing with a thin strip of thermoplastic dry bonded over the top.

MOULDING OVER JOINTS

Materials with a high degree of stretch and drape allow splints that traverse angulated joints to be

Figure 7 Creating holes. Once a hole is punched in the material, it can be gently stretched and rolled back until the desired size is achieved.

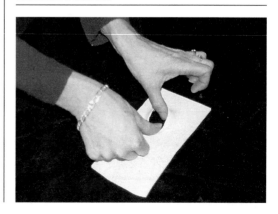

fabricated without seams to conform at the joint margins. The material is anchored either proximal or distal to the joint with a circumferential mould. The material can then be gently stretched over the joint, with the lateral aspects stretching less than the central aspect. This is particularly useful for elbow splints.

CIRCUMFERENTIAL SPLINTING

Materials that are self-adherent enable therapists to fabricate circumferential splints easily. A non-exact pattern is used, the material is pulled around the hand or arm and the edges lightly pinched together. No bandage or wrap is required as the material holds itself on the limb. This saves time, allowing the therapist to see and evaluate the splint easily whilst working. Bandaging is not required and this is beneficial for the patient who cannot tolerate a lot of handling. If the material is only lightly pinched together, it is easily pulled apart to release the patient. The splint may be finished either by hot seaming (e.g. cylindrical finger splint), by creating an opening where fasteners will be attached (e.g. circumferential wrist immobilizations splint), or both (e.g. hand-based thumb immobilization splint). Circumferential splints by

design are very strong and a thinner material can be used to achieve a high degree of rigidity and, therefore, immobility in the splinted part.

CUTTING THERMOPLASTIC MATERIAL

Shears are generally used to cut cold thermoplastics. Straight lines can be cut on sheets of thermoplastic by scoring it with a Stanley trimmer along a straight edge and then bending it to snap open the scored line. When cutting heated thermoplastics, use single, long strokes with scissors to ensure smooth edges. This is particularly important when cutting around curves.

ATTACHING STRAPS

Using adhesive-backed hook Velcro® is the easiest and quickest method to secure straps. Cut the Velcro® to the length required and round the corners. Ensure the area on the splint where Velcro® is to be attached is clean. Peel off the backing, heat the adhesive with a heat gun (hold the Velcro® with scissors or pliers to prevent injury) and attach to the splint at the correct location and angle. Press it on firmly ensuring there are no air bubbles. If this method is unsuccessful in securing the Velcro®, the surface of the thermoplastic can be spot heated with the heat gun, being careful not to distort it. The Velcro® is also heated and then pressed into place. Some materials with coating may require solvents or bonding agents to aid the process of adhering.

Splinting materials such as Orfit® and Aquaplast® can be heated until the surface is shiny, then the pile Velcro® applied directly to the material. Do not overheat the material or distort it with the pressure used to apply the strap. In materials where this is not possible, use hook Velcro® on both sides of the splint to attach the pile Velcro®.

In some materials, such as Hexcelite®, the adhesive will not remain secured to the splint. Attach the

Figure 8   Cutting hot seams. Pull the material around the limb and hold the edges together in a straight line. Using long scissor strokes, cut off the excess material as close to the limb as possible. A neat seam results.

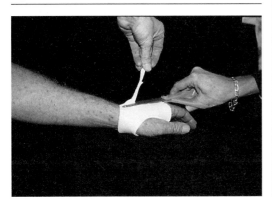

straps by adhering a piece of the material over the Velcro® or webbing. Best results are achieved if a small moon is cut from either side of the strap. Although this type of attachment is bulkier than a rivet, the advantage is that the inside surface of the orthosis remains smooth. This method is also useful when adhesive Velcro® and rivets are not available.

Stainless-steel rivets are rarely used owing to the efficiency of adhesive-backed Velcro®. They are time consuming, have a tendency to rust and require a riveter or hammer and anvil to secure them. If adhesive Velcro® is prohibitive (e.g. owing to cost), attach the Velcro® with as few rivets as possible and ensure placement allows flattening of the rivet completely on the surface against the skin to prevent pressure problems.

In some situations it may be necessary to consider using bandaging to secure the splint. For example, nursing home patients may have fragile skin intolerant of straps, may pick at and pull off the straps or injure themselves on the Velcro®, or pile straps may continually be lost.

D-rings may be used to make it easier for the patient to put on the splint, particularly when weakness is a problem. D-rings enable the patient to secure the splint more firmly. They are also useful where there is insufficient surface area on the splint to secure straps. The D-ring must be placed so its total surface is over the splint and not in contact with the skin.

APPLYING LINING

1. Apply all straps to the splint prior to lining it.
2. Retain the pattern from the splint and use it to outline the lining material. (Ensure the pattern is orientated so the adhesive back will adhere to the correct surface of the splint.)
3. For lining materials which have some 'give', allow approximately 1 cm around each edge, allow 2 cm for non-stretchable lining materials.

4. Apply the lining material to the splint in small sections. Do not take the whole backing sheet off at once.
5. Orientate the lining to the splint at the wrist and then work proximal and distal.
6. Avoid wrinkles or overlapping the lining material as this will cause pressure.
7. Trim the lining material to the edge of the splint, allowing a few millimetres overhang. Dry heating the exposed adhesive and adhering it over the edge of the splint prolongs the life of the lining.
8. The lining should be changed regularly as it becomes soiled.

Patient Preparation Procedures

INTRODUCTION

Discuss the purpose of the therapy session, the intended procedure and the expected outcomes, both short and long term. Clarify the patient's intended goals, and identify fears and anxieties. Inform the patient of expected pain or discomfort, e.g. if post-operative, the patient should expect some pain. Reassure the patient that the procedure itself should not cause pain. This is important as fear, anticipation of pain or lack of precautions can jeopardize the procedure. If the patient is a child, a few minutes spent at this point relaxing and having some fun, splinting the child's favourite doll or teddy, or letting them play with the thermoplastic material will save a lot of time later when an uninformed and tense child becomes non-compliant. If the child is unsettled, it is better to proceed as quickly and with as little fuss as possible.

A time frame for review of the splint is determined by the pathology and expected course of therapy intervention. Arrangements are necessary for after hours appointments or for referral to other practitioners where patients live far from the clinic.

EVALUATION

Obtain a complete clinical picture by thorough evaluation of the patient and their hand.

CLINICAL DECISION-MAKING

Decision-making is a collaborative effort between patient and therapist. Identify the therapy, and splinting requirements and objectives. Determine the extent of limb involvement and appropriate positions for joints involved in the splint. Identify design, material, strapping and lining options, and select the most suitable. Identify precautions for the therapist and the patient.

PATIENT INSTRUCTION

Describe the procedure of application and moulding of the splint and instruct the patient of the therapist's expectations of them during the procedure. (This includes where and how to hold the limb, and not to grasp the material unless asked to do so.) Advise the patient that the material should be warm but not hot.

ENVIRONMENT AND EQUIPMENT PREPARATION

Ensure the work area is clear of extraneous products. Wound dressings should be protected during splint fabrication or changed immediately after the splinting procedure. Gather all essential items and organize them in a tidy and accessible manner.

PATTERN TAKING

In order to create patterns, a therapist needs the ability to see a pattern in two dimensions transformed into a three-dimensional object. Take the pattern and ensure a correct fit before cutting it from the sheet of thermoplastic (Figure 9). Cut out the material and heat it.

PATIENT PREPARATION

While the material is heating, protect susceptible tissues. Pad out bony prominences and position the patient's limb for the splinting procedure. Small pieces of lining material or exercise putty can be moulded over protuberances prior to fabrication of the splint. Support tissues that are at risk, such as tendon repairs or metacarpophalangeal (MCP) arthroplasties. Protect grafts, flaps and pin sites.

SPLINT FABRICATION

Mould the splint according to requirements. Evaluate, check the position, fit and pressure, and correct or modify them as appropriate. Trim the excess, roll or smooth the edges, and apply the outriggers, straps and lining (if any).

Figure 9   Ensuring pattern fit. Line up the pattern landmarks with the underlying hand, and check the size and position.

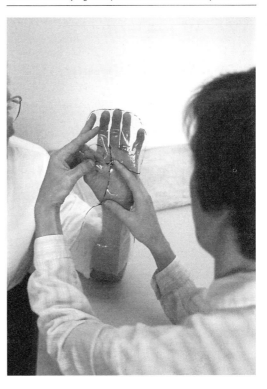

Place the splint back on the limb and conduct a final evaluation.

PATIENT EDUCATION

Educate the patient regarding wearing regimes, including the daily schedule, time span, weaning off, activities to avoid while wearing the splint, activities requiring removal of the splint and concomitant therapy requirements. Give the patient details about the care of the splint, including cleaning and protection from heat. Advise the patient to return if any problems are experienced (e.g. red areas, altered sensation, broken components) and inform the patient concerning follow-up or review appointments. The responsibility for the review process must be formalized (i.e. who is responsible for setting dates and conducting the review) with the therapist taking primary responsibility for his or her work. It is unethical to deliver treatment without some form of acceptable follow-up. It is advisable to issue a patient handout with all this information covered, including the therapist's name and a contact phone number.

RESTORATION OF THERAPEUTIC ENVIRONMENT

It is essential for safe and efficient work practices, let alone for professional presentation, to restore the environment to its original state. Clean and, if necessary, disinfect tools and equipment, and return them to the correct storage position.

Soiled towels and bandages should be stored for laundering, and fresh stocks replenished. Dressings, swabs and disposable packs should be disposed of appropriately. Surfaces should be cleaned of all waste materials and any water spills mopped up. Any stock re-ordering which is required should be noted.

Conclusion

Pride should be taken in all aspects of designing, fabricating and finishing off a splint. It represents visible evidence of the therapist's quality of work and will become part of the patient's personal presentation. If you would not like to be seen wearing it because it is unattractive, do not expect your patient to be compliant to the wearing regime. Quality fabrication is a result of sound knowledge of material characteristics and properties, and the ability to handle those materials to achieve maximum performance. As with the development of all technical skills, competency and efficiency is improved with practice. A well-organized, safe and efficient work environment assists in this process.

References

Breger-Lee, DE, Buford, WL (1992) Properties of thermoplastic splinting materials. *Journal of Hand Therapy* 5: 202–211.

Breger-Lee, DE (1995) Objective and subjective observations of low-temperature thermoplastic materials. *Journal of Hand Therapy* 8: 202–211.

4

Splinting to Address the Elbow and Forearm

Introduction

Normal use of the hand depends on a well-functioning elbow joint, as this is the critical link in lengthening and shortening the upper limb. Stability is crucial to ensure effective transmission of forces across the elbow joint. However, mobility is also important for function. Morrey *et al.* (1981) determined that normal functional range of elbow motion is 30°–130° with 100° rotation: 50° in supination and 50° pronation.

Anatomy of the Elbow and Forearm

The elbow complex consists of the ulnohumeral and the radiohumeral articulations, with close associations to the proximal radioulnar (PRU) joint. Whilst commonly considered a hinge joint, owing to its primary motion of flexion–extension, accessory movements of abduction, adduction and axial rotation are well recognized (Morrey and Chao, 1976). The centre of rotation of the elbow remains an issue of discussion with most authors agreeing that there are centres of rotation, which correspond to a line from the inferior aspect of the medial epicondyle through the centre of the lateral epicondyle (An and Morrey, 1993; Werner and An, 1994).

The obliquities between the proximal humeral shaft, the trochlea and the distal ulna shaft define the carrying angle. In the frontal plane, this valgus angle averages 10°–15° in men and 15°–20° in women; however, the angle is not evident in pronation. The changes in the carrying angle, from extension to flexion in the frontal plane, are still debated in the literature (Youm et al., 1979; London, 1981; Morrey, 1985) (Figure 1). The clinical implication pertains to the use of articulated splints. The axis of motion of the elbow and the

degree of rotation of the forearm, and the alignment of the axis of the hinge require careful attention to avoid misalignment.

Stability is afforded to the joint by the congruous articular surfaces and the soft tissue constraints. The trochlear notch of the olecranon articulates with the conical trochlea of the humerus and is the primary determinant of bony stability. The radiohumeral joint also contributes to lateral stability and force transmission through the elbow. The ulnohumeral, radiohumeral and PRU joints are enclosed within a common fibrous capsule. This is reinforced by the medial and lateral collat-

Figure 1 Changes in the carrying angle of the forearm. Changes in the carrying angle are seen as the radius rotates in relation to the ulna from supination (a) to pronation (b) (reproduced from Kapandji, 1982, p. 113 with permission), and from a vaglus angle in elbow extension to a varus angle in elbow flexion (reproduced from Morrey and Chao, 1975, p. 503).

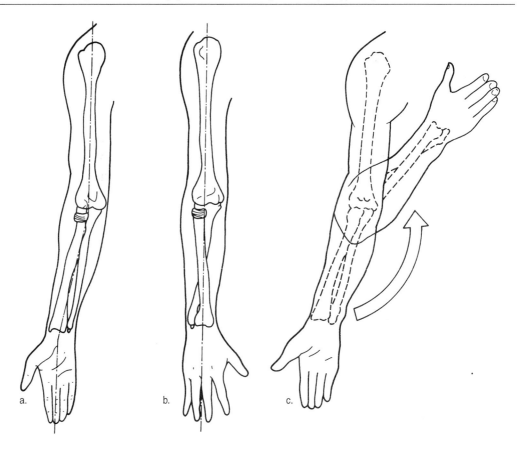

eral ligaments. Of these, the medial ligament is the most important owing to the orientation of functional stress. The medial collateral ligament consists of anterior and posterior bundles that contribute to stability in different ranges of motion (Regan *et al.*, 1991). The flexor pronator muscles also contribute to stability. The lateral collateral ligament is more variable with the majority of fibres attaching to the annular ligament. The anconeous muscle contributes to lateral stability along with wrist and finger extensor musculature.

Whilst functionally distinct joints, the proximity of the ulnohumeral to the radiohumeral and to the proximal radioulnar joints implies that injury to one joint may have consequences for the mobility of the others.

Rotary motion occurs at the proximal and distal radioulnar joints in the actions of pronation and supination. The axis of rotation is through the centre of the radial head and capitulum, and along the line extending through the base of the ulna styloid (Figure 2). While most authors agree that the radius rotates in an arc around the ulna during pronation–supination, the contribution of the ulna to this movement is still an area for discussion. The two radioulnar joints are coaxial. While greater motion is seen at the distal joint as the radius rotates about the ulna, it must be remembered that, except when either of the bones is malaligned, the radius rotates through the same arc of motion at the PRU and distal radioulnar (DRU) joints. Wrist and hand splints applied to a forearm surface must allow for the changing dimensions of the forearm during rotation (Figure 3). Pronation supination is easily compromised by fractures of the radius and ulna. Maximizing the range of the forearm rotation is a therapeutic goal commonly addressed by splinting.

Figure 2   Axis of motion for pronation–supination. This axis is located along the entire length of the forearm. Traction applied at a 90° angle could approximate a 360° curve (from Colello-Abraham, 1990, p. 1135).

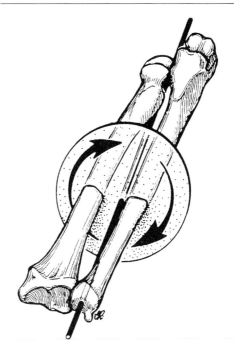

Rotation of the head of the radius about its axis occurs within the fibro-osseous ring formed by the annular ligament and the radial notch of the ulna. The unique shape of the proximal radius and the head of the radius means that rotatory movements are also accompanied by lateral movement and distal tilting of the radius. The flexibility in the annular ligament permits this movement.

The DRU joint is the head of the ulna articulating on the concave sigmoid notch of the radius. While the joint surfaces are well adapted to each other, the joint geometry varies with the relative length of the ulna to the radius. Stability of the distal joint is due to the triangular fibrocartilage complex (TFCC), the radioulnar ligaments, and the capsule (see Figure 1 of Chapter 5). The TFCC consists of a cartilaginous central portion

Figure 3   Changing shape and orientation of the forearm on rotation. Longitudinal lines the length of the forearm illustrate the changes in alignment and orientation from supination to pronation.

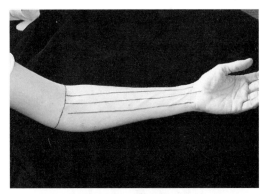

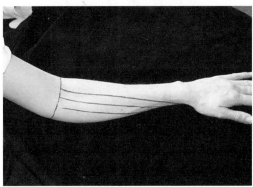

(the disc), surrounded by thick dorsal and volar radioulnar ligaments, the ulnar collateral ligament, the meniscus homologue, the extensor carpi ulnaris sheath, the ulnolunate and lunotriquetral ligaments. Translocation of the ulna, dorsally during pronation and volarly during supination, is checked by the dorsal and volar DRU joint ligaments thus preventing dislocation. Instability, impingement and incongruity are common problems of the DRU joint, which impact on the functional range available for rotation. The midcarpal joint is isolated from the radiocarpal joint, except when there are deficits in the triangular fibrocartilage secondary to trauma or degeneration.

Tremendous forces are transmitted across the elbow joint by the action of powerful flexor and extensor muscles. Elbow flexion is achieved by biceps brachii, brachialis and brachioradialis with triceps the extensor. Brachialis muscle is implicated in post-traumatic contracture of the elbow owing to its location on the anterior capsule of the elbow. Haematoma in the muscle is an inciting cause of heterotopic ossification (deposition of calcium within the muscle) and subsequent capsular contracture (Weiss and Sachar, 1994).

Laterally the wrist and hand extensor musculature arise from the supracondylar ridge and lateral epicondyle. Medially the flexor pronator group arise from the medial epicondyle. By their location proximal to the elbow joint, the wrist extensor and flexor musculature have a small moment arm for rotation at the elbow, but a significant contribution to joint stability. Epicondylitis, a common clinical presentation with pain in the region of either the medial or lateral epicondyle, is exacerbated by resisted action of muscles arising from the involved epicondyle.

The major nerves to the hand traverse the elbow joint and, with the exception of the ulnar nerve, are generally protected by the muscles through which they traverse. Attention should be focused on the ulnar nerve, in its path around the medial epicondyle, to ensure that it is not compromised by pressure from any form of splint intervention.

Splints Designed to Immobilize the Elbow

Immobilization of the elbow can be achieved with or without immobilization of forearm rotation.

Figure 4 Elbow splint pattern. Location of the circumferential and length measurements required to make a pattern for an elbow splint.

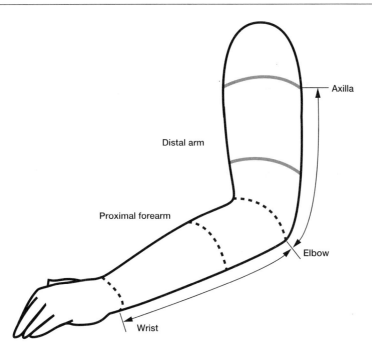

Circumferential designs offer the greatest immobilization and are required following some injuries in the vicinity of the elbow, while posterior application is recommended for splints to immobilize the elbow for rest.

Splints to address the elbow (Figures 5 and 6) use a series of length and circumferential measurements as illustrated in Figure 4.

Elbow Immobilization Splint (Anterior or Posterior Surface) (Figures 6 and 7)

When the elbow is immobilized at angles less than 70° flexion, the property of stretch and mould are used to contour the material to the arm. However, if the angle is greater than 70° flexion, a dart must be taken out of the splinting material at the elbow to ensure contour.

Numerous bony prominences require padding prior to fabrication. Where the biceps muscle is also tight, as in the case of an elbow contracture, care should be taken to avoid pressure on the tendon.

Measurements required for this splint are taken with the arm in the position in which it will be splinted (see Figure 5):

1 Length axilla—elbow—wrist proximal to the ulna head.
2 Circumference at the axilla.
3 Circumference at the wrist proximal to the ulna head.
4 Circumference proximal to the elbow (one third the length measurement of the upper arm).
5 Circumference below the elbow (one third the length measurement of the forearm).

Figure 5   Posterior elbow immobilization splint. This splint is generally used to rest and support the soft tissues.

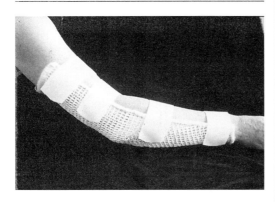

Figure 6   Anterior elbow immobilization splint. Splints applied to the anterior surface minimize the risk of pressure problems at the elbow; however, they require circumferential strapping to maintain position, particularly when used with persons with elbow spasticity.

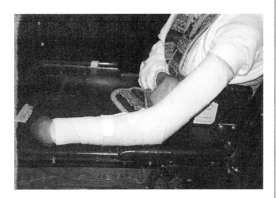

PROCEDURE TO MAKE A PATTERN

1. Draw a vertical line in the centre of your pattern material the length of the arm (Figure 7).

2. Square three lines through this at the level of the axilla, elbow and wrist. Mark the points where the circumferences were taken proximal to the elbow and proximal forearm, then insert the related circumferences. For circumferential splints, use the full measurement, with two thirds the measurement for anterior or posterior splints.

3. Darts may be required in splints applied to the posterior surface. In that case, mark the depth of two 'V-shaped' darts at the elbow (see Figure 8, inset).

4. Cut one side of the dart. The triangles at the edges of the dart are brought together. The overlap material is used to reinforce the bond.

5. Apply the pattern to the patient's arm, make any adjustment to the pattern prior to transferring it to the splinting material.

FABRICATION PROCEDURE

Owing to the large piece of splinting material involved in this pattern, some planning is required to avoid difficulties. When removing the material from the heating pan, ensure that it is supported along the length to avoid stretching. Anterior application is easiest by placing the material on the arm aligning the elbow crease with the elbow component. For posterior application, it may be easier to lie the patient down, either supine or prone, and use shoulder movement to position the arm and forearm so that gravity can be used to assist application. For circumferential splints, apply the anterior surface then bring the posterior component around to bond on either the medial or lateral borders.

The type of splinting material has implications to fabrication technique. Non-stick materials are easier to handle in large pieces; however, they require the additional step of bandaging to secure the material to the limb. An assistant may be required or the patient instructed how to assist. Classic Orfit® must be handled with care so that it does not inadvertently stick to itself but has the great advantage of sticking to the patient's limb, thereby eliminating the need to bandage.

Figure 8   Elbow immobilization splint pattern.

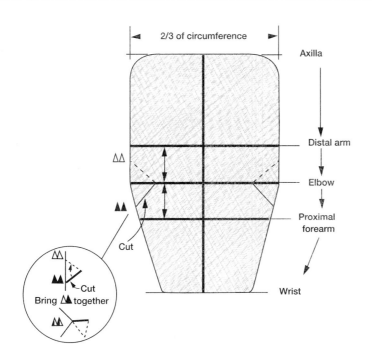

Splints Designed to Mobilize the Elbow

Deficits in passive range of motion of the elbow, particularly extension, are a common complication of injury to the joint and surrounding soft tissues. The high propensity for contracture, even following relatively minor trauma, increases the importance of prevention. Forceful manipulation of the joint can be counterproductive by tearing tissue and stimulating further contracture. Therefore, by applying a small force to extend the tissues for a prolonged period of time by using mobilizing splints, gradual lengthening of tissues can be achieved. Resolution of elbow contractures may take many months of splint application so

determining the commitment of the patient is essential prior to undertaking splint fabrication.

Numerous designs are used to address the flexion contracture of the elbow. Static progressive splints are the most effective. However, where a hinge would pose a risk, as with young children or those persons with altered cognitive abilities, serial static designs are recommended.

Hinged Elbow Mobilizing Splint

Static progressive splints are a cost-effective means of addressing elbow contractures. Although the hinges are expensive, they can be adjusted as the joint accommodates to changes in range of motion (ROM). If the patient is responsible, he or she may be educated to do this, thereby reducing the cost of consultation with the therapist.

PATTERN AND FABRICATION PROCEDURE

Hinged elbow splints as illustrated in Figure 8 require circumferential cuffs for the arm and forearm.

1. Length and circumferential measurements are taken using locations identified in Figure 4.
2. Cuffs are made and two straps are attached to each cuff. Cuffs are fitted to the arm and forearm prior to application of the hinge.
3. Alignment of the hinge axis to the axis of the elbow is determined. Mark the location of the attachment of the hinge to the arm cuff.
4. Secure the hinge to the cuff with an additional piece of thermoplastic material. Fit the arm cuff with the attached hinge, align the axes of the hinge and the joint, then carefully mark the location for bonding the hinge to the forearm cuff. Secure the hinge with a second bond.
5. Apply the splint to the arm and check the hinge

Figure 8   Hinged elbow splint. Alignment of the axis and arms of the hinge to the axis of the joint, and the humerus and ulna are critical to maximize torque. Screws allow for adjustment of the joint position or restriction of the joint range.

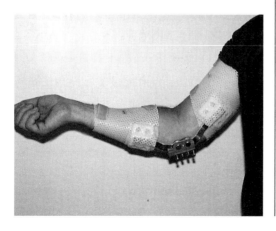

alignment and also all edges. Flare all edges to ensure there is no shear pressure.

6. If the patient is to modify the hinge angle himself or herself, he or she must be instructed in the following:

(a) When to wear the splint. This will be determined by lifestyle. Some patients are better able to tolerate the splint during the day whilst others can comfortably wear the splint during sleep. Prior to wearing this splint during sleep, the patient should have worn it for extended periods during the day to ensure no complications.

(b) When to change the angle. This will be determined by compliance of tissues to lengthen in response to the gentle stress applied. It is recommended that patients wear the splint for upwards of 6 hours per day for several days with 'no awareness of pulling or tension in the tissues' before increasing the passive range by several degrees.

(c) The procedure to change the angle. It is important that the patient has the necessary tools and has demonstrated competence in the procedure prior to leaving the clinic.

(d) Precautions. Attempting to increase the angle faster than the tissues can accommodate may result in injury to tissue and further scarring. The patient must understand the risks of incorrect use of the splint.

Serial Static Elbow Mobilizing Splint

The design found to be most effective to address deficits in extension ROM involves a circumferential component around the arm with an ante-

Figure 9   Serial static elbow splint. The circumferential arm component provides extensive anchorage and pressure distribution. This design is commonly used with children.

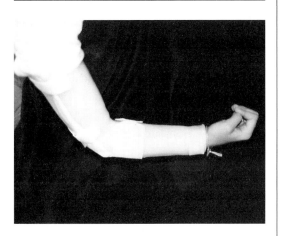

rior component around the forearm (Figure 9). If forearm rotation is not an issue, then position the forearm in supination or pronation as muscle and subcutaneous tissue will disperse the pressure. This design requires frequent remoulding and, therefore, it should be made of splinting material that has a memory to accommodate changes over time.

PROCEDURE TO TAKE A PATTERN

The measurements required for the pattern are taken in locations marked in Figure 4. Full circumferential measurements are used for the arm and two thirds measurements for the forearm as illustrated in Figure 10.

When the patient has to apply this splint, the opening is located on the medial aspect of the arm. However, when easy access to the straps is not desirable, as may be the case for young children, the opening may be located on the lateral surface. If an assistant is able to hold the limb in the desired extended position, the splint can be made in one moulding.

FABRICATION PROCEDURE

1. The splinting material is carefully removed from the heating source and applied to the limb bonding the medial edges of the arm component. Splinting materials that do not adhere to themselves will require bandaging.
2. Gentle force is applied to place tissues at the end of their passive range and sustained until the material is totally cold.
3. Mark any modifications.
4. All edges are heated, smoothed and flared away from the skin.
5. Straps are applied to secure the arm and forearm components.

The splint can also be moulded in two stages. This is best achieved by softening the required region, then softening to a lessor extent an additional region 4–5 cm wide. (A single line demarcating heated and non-heated material cannot be well controlled.)

1. Heat the splinting material. The arm component material is fully activated whilst the forearm component remains only partially softened.
2. Apply to the arm, moulding to ensuring good contour. The elbow need only be positioned.
3. Complete the fabrication of the arm component, curving the proximal edge and apply the straps.
4. Reheat the forearm component just past the elbow.
5. Apply the hard arm component to the limb securing the straps, then apply gentle pressure to extend the elbow whilst moulding the elbow region and forearm component.
6. Complete the fabrication of the forearm component, curve the edges and apply the straps.

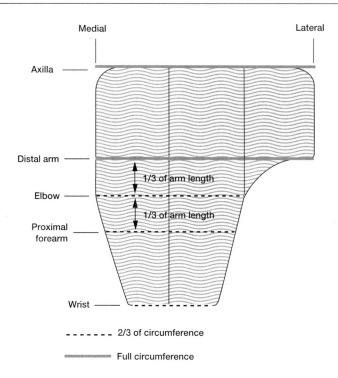

Figure 10   Serial static elbow splint pattern.

Splints Designed to Immobilize the Forearm

Complete immobilization of the forearm can only be achieved when both proximal and distal joints are addressed. For this reason it is necessary to include the wrist and the distal humerus. Thus splints that immobilize the forearm generally immobilize the wrist and restrict motion at the elbow.

Splints that immobilize the forearm present a unique challenge (Figures 11 and 13). The therapist must manage large pieces of splinting material whilst controlling multiple joints. To achieve the desired function of the splint, the therapist must control the position of the wrist, forearm and the elbow during moulding. To simplify this process, a splint is described which is made in two stages. The two-stage design is also recommended if the patient has a lot of pain and/or if greater care is required during the moulding process. An alternative design that traverses the volar and dorsal surfaces of the hand and forearm whilst allowing elbow flexion, is more suited to rigid materials that have to be bandaged on to the forearm. The bandaging process requires great care so that the forearm is not rotated when circumferentially wrapping the splint to the forearm.

Forearm Immobilization Splint

The design incorporates the landmarks for the volar and dorsal wrist immobilization splints (Figure 12). However, placement of the hand on the table to take a pattern will require too much

Figure 12   Forearm immobilization splint. This splint is circumferential in the distal forearm and wrist (top). Allowance is made on the anterior surface at the proximal end for some degree of active elbow flexion (bottom).

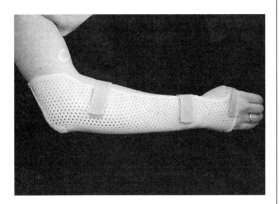

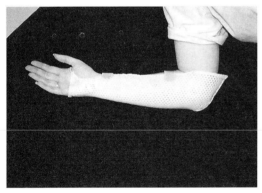

rotation, therefore, the arm is supported at the elbow and pattern material wrapped around volar and dorsal surfaces.

PROCEDURE TO MAKE A PATTERN

Mark the following points as illustrated in Figure 12:

1 Lateral aspects of the hand just proximal to the heads of the index finger metacarpal on the volar and dorsal surfaces.

2 Radial aspect of the hand at the thumb web level.

3 Ulnar aspect of the hand proximal to the head of the little finger metacarpal.

4 Lateral aspect of the wrist at mid-carpal level on the volar and dorsal surfaces. This will indicate wrist circumference.

5 The elbow crease on the anterior surface. This will indicate proximal forearm circumference.

6 Posterior aspect of the arm at the same level as point 5 taking into account the distal arm circumference. This point also determines the length of the splint.

7 The olecranon.

8 Tip of the middle finger.

9 Webspace between the index and middle fingers on the volar and dorsal surfaces.

To shape the pattern:

1. Join points 1 and 3 (MCP line).

2. On the volar surface, draw a vertical line from point 8 to the level of the wrist. Draw a vertical line from point 9 to the level of the MCP line, this is point 10. These lines are used as a guide to the thenar eminence.

3. Starting at point 10, draw a line to following the thenar crease around to the wrist at point 4.

4. On the dorsal surfaces, draw a vertical line from point 9 to the level of the wrist.

5. On the dorsal surface shape the line from point 2 to follow the thenar eminence around to the wrist at point 4.

6. Join points 4, 5 and 6, and then sharply curve around to point 7.

7. Cut the pattern out and check for fit on the patient, prior to transferring it to the thermoplastic material. Materials that use a gravity assist to facilitate moulding are not recommended for these splints. Owing to the large area of the forearm covered in splinting material, perforations are also recommended.

FABRICATION PROCEDURE

1. The arm should be positioned so that it is supported with clearance under the elbow, the

Figure 12   Pattern for a forearm immobilization splint. The dorsal and volar wrist immobilization splint patterns are combined to immobilize the forearm and lengthened to accommodate the elbow.

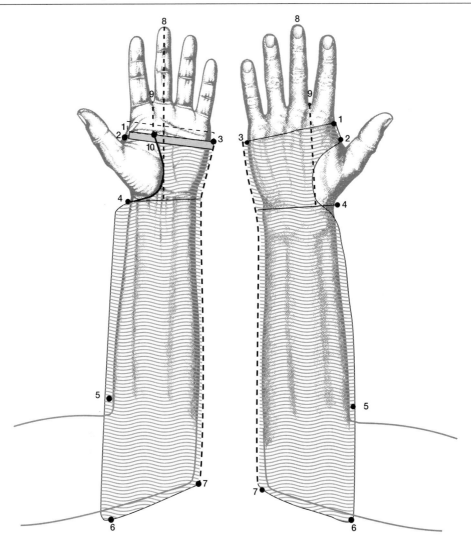

forearm in a vertical position in the desired position of rotation and the wrist in the predetermined position. Pad out the ulna head and all bony prominences around the elbow prior to fabrication.

2. Remove the thermoplastic material from the heating source taking care to support the length of the material so that it does not stretch. Apply to the hand bonding volar and dorsal components through the webspace and along the radial aspect of the forearm.

3. Now bond the material on the posterior aspect of the elbow. Cut this seam hot for a smooth seam.

4. Ensure the position of forearm rotation is maintained, and the material is well contoured

through the arches of the hand and around the wrist.

5. When completely cold, mark the edges that need to be rolled, then remove the splint from the arm.

6. Add an extra piece of material to seal the posterior elbow seam.

7. Very gently reheat the edges and roll. Ensure clearance for movement of the fingers at the MCP joints, the thenar eminence and some degrees of elbow flexion. The rolled edge decreases shear stress and improves comfort whilst also providing reinforcement.

8. Attach three straps, one at each end of the forearm, and one through the thumb webspace.

This design allows elbow flexion greater than 90°. Deficits in elbow extension common on removing the splint are resolved with active and passive movement.

Forearm Immobilization Splint – Two-Stage Fabrication

The design uses a long circumferential wrist immobilization splint with an additional component added to the anterior surface to enclose the anterior, medial and lateral surfaces of the elbow and arm completely (Figure 13). The posterior aspect is free, which allows the patient to remove the wide straps and carefully range the elbow into extension. If complete immobilization of the elbow is necessary, the arm component is made circumferential.

Wrist and forearm immobilization is a common requirement following injury to the distal radius and ulna. The duration of immobilization of the forearm is often less than that for the wrist, therefore, this design accommodates that change. An additional advantage of this design is that, if defi-

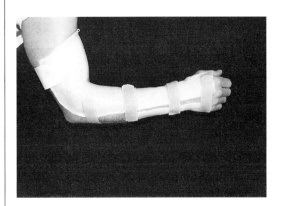

Figure 13 Forearm immobilization splint – two-stage fabrication. Prevention of forearm rotation is achieved by extending a circumferential wrist immobilization splint on the anterior surface of the arm.

cits in pronation or supination exist after the period of immobilization, the wrist immobilization splint can be easily incorporated into a forearm mobilizing splint.

To make this splint, use the pattern and fabrication instructions for the circumferential wrist immobilization splint (Figure 15 on page 99). Increase the length of the forearm so that the proximal end finishes distal to the elbow crease. The opening of the wrist splint may be either dorsal or dorsal ulnar. Complete the fabrication excluding rolling the proximal end on the anterior surface and attaching the proximal strap.

The size of the piece of material to extend the splint past the elbow is determined by three measurements:

1 Length from proximal end of the splint to the level of the axilla on the anterior aspect of the arm.

2 Distal width is from medial epicondyle around the anterior aspect of the elbow to the lateral epicondyle.

3 Proximal width is two-thirds the circumference of the arm at the level of the axilla.

The forearm is positioned in the desired position of rotation with the wrist immobilization splint *in situ*. Pad out the bony prominences around the elbow prior to fabrication. The arm piece is heated then positioned to overlap the splint by approximately 2 cm and moulded around the anterior surface of the arm ensuring good contour along the medial and lateral aspects of the elbow. When cold, the join between the two splint components is reheated to ensure a solid bond. The proximal end is flared. The third strap for the forearm component is attached along with a wide strap proximal on the arm component.

If the pathology is located in the distal radioulnar joint, the deficits in elbow flexion common on removal of this type of splint are resolved over several weeks with functional movement and passive exercise.

Splints Designed to Mobilize the Forearm

Deficits in supination of the forearm present a greater functional limitation than deficits in pronation. Abduction and internal rotation of the shoulder will compensate for pronation. However, no other movement can substitute for supination.

Splint choices to mobilize the forearm in directions of pronation and supination include a custom-made serial progressive splint, a dynamic splint (Colello-Abraham, 1990) and a variety of prefabricated splints (Figure 14). In preformed splints (Rolyan®), tension is created by torsional bars that apply force in oblique directions to the

axis of rotation from an elbow component to a hand component.

Rotation of the forearm occurs at the coaxial proximal and distal radioulnar joints. The axis of rotation of the forearm is found the length of the radius and ulna. A force applied at any point along the length of these bones to effect rotation will affect both joints equally.

The design for a serial progressive splint is simple to make and has high patient acceptance in comparison to other designs. It consists of an anterior

Figure 14   Forearm mobilizing splints. (top) A serial progressive splint combines a circumferential wrist immobilization splint and an anterior elbow immobilization splint with force applied by a Velcro® strap. (bottom) A dynamic pronation–supination splint applies force via a wrist immobilization splint from an aluminium frame in clockwise or counter clockwise directions to effect rotation of the forearm.

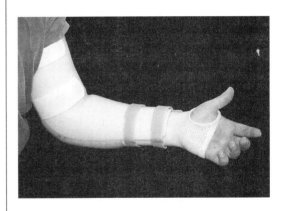

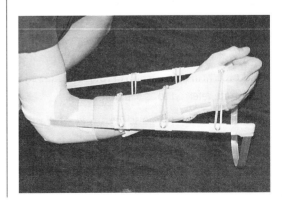

elbow immobilization splint and a circumferential wrist immobilization splint. To create torque that maximizes the rotatory component, force is applied perpendicular to the axis of motion. As forearm rotation normally occurs in a circular motion through approximately 180°, traction can be applied to effect a rotary torque at any point through this arc. The area of force application is determined by the size of the wrist immobilization splint. The hand is included in the forearm splint as much of the pathology affecting forearm rotation also has an impact upon the wrist. Also, inclusion of the hand increases the area for distal anchorage and patient comfort.

FABRICATION PROCEDURE

1. Make a circumferential wrist immobilization splint (instructions for the pattern and fabrication procedures are found on page 99).
2. Make an anterior elbow immobilization splint (instructions for the pattern and fabrication procedures are found on page 71). When moulding this splint, just prior to the material becoming completely hard, slightly increase the circumference of the forearm component to allow for the wrist immobilization splint underneath. Secure the straps to the arm component.
3. Attach two pieces of adhesive-backed hook Velcro® in a circumferential direction to the wrist immobilization splint, one at the wrist and the other at the mid-forearm level. A long piece of pile Velcro® is then attached, wrapping around the forearm in the direction of rotation required. These are referred to as rotation straps.

   Rotation straps may also be made of elastic Velcro® or 25 mm woven elastic band with a piece of pile Velcro® sewn to each end.
4. Secure the elbow splint in place. Take the rotation strap on the wrist splint and wrap it around

over the anterior surface of the elbow splint. Mark the location and then apply the adhesive-backed hook Velcro®.

To use the splint, the patient takes the rotation straps, rotates the forearm in the direction of the deficit to end range and then secures them to the elbow splint. The forearm is now held at the end range of motion. As the tissues accommodate the position, the rotation straps can be altered to increase the degree of rotation.

Experience has shown, as with many other joints, that wearing tolerance to this serial progressive splint is generally much longer than that for the dynamic splint. The advantages of this splint are its ease and speed of fabrication, its acceptance by patients owing to its appearance and its ease of application.

Detailed procedures to fabricate a dynamic pronation–supination splint (Figure 14b) are described by Collelo-Abraham (1990). Aesthetics of this splint, as well as ease of fabrication, are increased considerably by the use of aluminium rod and dressmaking coat hooks.

Other Elbow Splints

Splints used to address the symptoms of lateral epicondylitis are in a unique category. They are designed to reduce the stresses on the common forearm extensor muscle origin. The splint consists of an non-elastic band several centimetres wide, which is secured by a Velcro® strap looped through a 'D' ring (Figure 15). Several brands are available from splinting material suppliers and retail through pharmacies. It is proposed that the band provides a counterforce to the forearm musculature, decreasing the capacity of the mus-

Figure 15 Lateral epicondylitis splint. This circumferential splint is applied distal to the elbow.

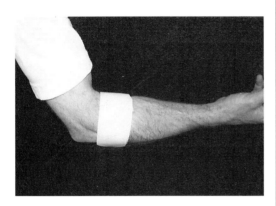

cles to contract, thereby decreasing the stress on the injured muscle fibres (Groppel and Nirschl, 1986; Wadsworth *et al.*, 1989; Wright and Rettig, 1995). The literature reports wide variability in the success of splints to address the symptoms of localized pain in the region of the lateral epicondyle of the humerus, and strength of grip and functional tasks due to pain with attempted muscle function (Clementis and Chow, 1993; Groppel and Nirschl, 1986). The criterion for prescription of counterforce splints for persons with lateral epicondylitis is based on subjective symptoms of pain and impaired function. Modification of symptoms may result from wearing the splint; however, it is vital that the cause of the problem and the biomechanics of loading forearm musculature are addressed in relation to vocational or recreational demands.

Conclusion

The elbow and forearm provide important freedoms of movement to the upper limb. Orientation of the hand, with sufficient functional motion towards the face and away from the body can be achieved by tissues that allow motion through the majority of the available range. Whilst numerous splints are manufactured to rest structures to allow healing, by far the greater role of splinting in both the elbow and forearm is maximizing the recovery of range of motion.

References

An, KN, Morrey, BF (1993) Biomechanics of the elbow. In: Morrey, BF (ed) *The Elbow and its Disorders*, 2nd edn, pp. 53–72. Philadelphia: WB Saunders.

Clementis, LG, Chow, S (1993) Effectiveness of a custom-made below elbow lateral counter force splint in the treatment of lateral epicondylitis. *Canadian Journal of Occupational Therapy* **60**: 137–144.

Colello-Abraham, K (1990) Dynamic pronation–supination splint. In: Hunter, JM, Schneider, LH, Makin, EJ, Callahan, AD (eds) *Rehabilitation of the Hand: Surgery and Therapy*, 3rd edn, pp. 1134–1139. St Louis: Mosby.

Groppel, J, Nirschl, R (1986) A mechanical and electromyographical analysis of the effects of various counterforce braces on the tennis player. *American Journal of Sports Medicine* **14**: 195–200.

Kapandji, IA (1982) *The Physiology of the Joints. Volume I. Upper Limb*. Edinburgh: Churchill Livingstone.

London, JT (1981) Kinematics of the elbow. *Journal of Bone and Joint Surgery* **63A**: 529–535.

Morrey, BF (1985) Functional anatomy in mechanics of the elbow. In: Kashiwagi, D (ed) *Elbow Joint*, pp. 295–303. Amsterdam: Elsevier Science Publishers.

Morrey, BF, Chao, EYS (1976) Passive motion of the elbow joint. *Journal of Bone and Joint Surgery* **58A**: 501–508.

Morrey, BF, Askew, LJ, An, KN (1981) A biomechanical study of normal functional elbow motion. *Journal of Bone and Joint Surgery* **63A**: 872–877.

Regan, WD, Korinek, SL, Morrey, BF, An, KN (1991) Biomechanical study of the ligaments around the elbow joint. *Clinical Orthopaedics and Related Research* **271**: 170–179.

Wadsworth, C, Neilsen, D, Burns, L, *et al.* (1989) Effect of the counterforce armband on wrist extension and grip strength and pain in subjects with tennis elbow. *Journal of Orthopedics and Sports Physiotherapy* **11**: 192–197.

Weiss, AC, Sachar, K (1994) Soft tissue contractures about the elbow. *Hand Clinics* **10**: 439–451.

Werner, FW, An, KN (1994) Biomechanics of the elbow and forearm. *Hand Clinics* **10**: 357–373.

Wright, HH, Rettig, AC (1995) Management of common sports injuries. In: Hunter, JM, Makin, EJ, Callahan, AD (eds) *Rehabilitation of the Hand: Surgery and Therapy*, 4th edn, pp. 1809–1838. St Louis: Mosby.

Youm, Y, Dwyer, RF, Thambyrajah, K, *et al.* (1979) Biomechanical analysis of the forearm pronation–supination and elbow flexion–extension. *Journal of Biomechanics* **12**: 245–255.

5

Splinting to Address the Wrist and Hand

Introduction
•
Anatomy of the Wrist and Hand
•
Splints Designed to Immobilize the Wrist and Hand
•
Splints Designed to Mobilize the Wrist
•
Splint Designed to Restrict Motion in the Wrist
•
Conclusion

Introduction

The wrist is often described as the key to hand function as it provides a mobile yet stable base for the fingers and the thumb that is independent of forearm position. The challenge for the therapist is to restore function in the wrist where normal biomechanical relationships are disrupted as a result of injury or disease affecting bones, joints, ligaments and muscles. Splinting is often the treatment intervention chosen to achieve this objective. This chapter will specifically address splints fabricated for the wrist and include a splint to rest the whole hand. Splints that include the wrist, where the primary function is to address pathol-

ogy at the distal radioulnar joint, the fingers or thumb, are described in the chapters that address those regions.

Anatomy of the Wrist and Hand

This short review of anatomy of the wrist and hand is intended to highlight critical issues of anatomy that impact upon the design and fabrication of the splints for this region. Of particular interest is the architectural arrangement of the bones and formation of arches, the inter-relationship between extrinsic and intrinsic musculature to effect motion of the wrist and fingers, and the soft tissue coverings of skin and fascia. Wrist anatomy and biomechanics in health and disease remain an area of much discussion amongst anatomists, surgeons and therapists.

Dysfunction in the wrist is common following disruption of articular surfaces and ligaments resulting in deformity, instability and loss of motion. Restoration of normal anatomy and biomechanics is not possible for many patients. Therefore, knowledge of normal anatomy and kinesiology is essential to understanding the changes that have occurred in the injured wrist, whilst an understanding of pathology is essential to determine the appropriate course of therapy intervention.

Architecture and Structure

Splinting the wrist to rest, position, or to regain mobility requires knowledge of the relationships formed by different skeletal structures· of the hand (Berger and Garcia-Elias, 1991). Motion results from the interactions of the carpal bones between themselves, as well as proximally with the articulating surface of the radius and the ulna/ triangular fibrocartilage complex, and distally with the bases of the metacarpals. The shape of the articulating surfaces of the carpals combines with strong ligamentous connections to control motion created by muscles that generally insert distal to the joint.

Functionally, the carpals may be considered in proximal and distal rows. The distal carpals have interlocking articular surfaces between themselves and the index and middle finger metacarpals. Thus, the magnitude and direction of movement of the index and middle finger metacarpals is reflected in motion of the distal carpals (Berger, 1996). The movement of the proximal row is a lot more variable; however, these carpals also tend to function as a unit. The scaphoid spanning both carpal rows plays a critical role in providing stability to what is an inherently unstable arrangement. The inter-relationships between the carpals as the wrist moves through the ranges of flexion and extension, and radial and ulnar deviation, are very complex. While the theories that attempt to explain this phenomenon are beyond the scope of this review, the therapist is encouraged to consider the complexity of joint and ligamentous arrangements, particularly when designing splints to mobilize the wrist joint.

The articular surface of the distal radius faces ulnarly at an angle of approximately 15° and this means that the axis of flexion–extension is oblique to the axis of the forearm. The wrist normally rests in a few degrees of ulnar deviation, with greater range of motion in ulnar deviation as compared to radial deviation. The articular surface also has a slightly volar tilt contributing to slightly greater motion in flexion than extension. The restraining influence of the ligaments of the radiocarpal and mid-carpal joints (Figure 1), the retinacular ligaments of the wrist combined with the wrist muscles, and the agonist antagonist balance of the extrinsic and intrinsic finger muscles, dictate the normal resting positions of wrist and hand joints. These factors also determine joint interaction in functional patterns of motion.

Movement of the wrist occurs about the axes of flexion and extension, and radial and ulnar deviation. Functionally, movements are also seen in the direction of extension radial deviation and flexion ulnar deviation. The centre of rotation of these axes is considered to be the head of the capitate (Berger, 1996). Thus, when a hinged or articulated wrist splint is required, alignment of the axis of wrist motion to the axis of the splint hinge is critical. However, it must be remembered that

Figure 1   The wrist ligaments. Dissection and illustration showing ligaments which constrain, and thus influence, radiocarpal and intercarpal motion. (a) Dorsal ligaments; (b) volar ligaments. RS, radioscaphoid; RT, radiotriquetral; TFCC, triangular fibrocartilage complex; DIC, dorsal intercarpal ligaments; RCL, radial collateral ligament; RC, radiocapitate; C, capitate; T, triquetrum; RSL, radioscapholunate; ECU sheath, extensor carpi ulnaris sheath; UT, ulnotriquetral; UL, ulnolunate; TFC, triangular fibrocartilage. Reproduced from Palmer (1988, pp. 993 and 994).

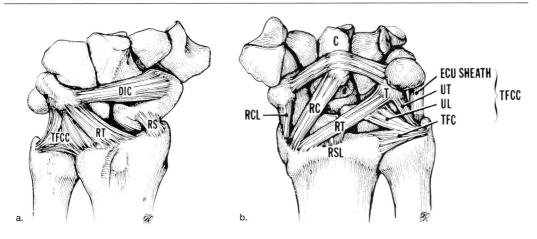

Figure 2   The arches of the hand. The longitudinal and transverse arches of the hand are shown in a side view. The shaded areas show the fixed part of the skeleton. Reproduced from Tubiana (1981, p. 25).

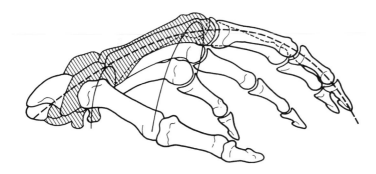

hinges have only one axis of motion, thus any deviation associated with flexion and extension is eliminated.

Fractures of the distal radius and carpals, along with tendon and muscle injury result in swelling and fibrosis that can severely compromise wrist movement. Thus, the position in which the joint is immobilized to allow healing must account for an outcome of stiffness and limited motion, and consider how this position may have an affect on the functional use of the hand.

The skeleton of the hand is composed of fixed elements of the distal row of carpals and the index and middle finger metacarpals, surrounded by the other mobile elements of the proximal carpal row and the metacarpals of the thumb, ring and little fingers, and the phalanges to all digits. The architectural arrangement of bones forms a series of arches (Figures 2 and 3). Transverse arches exist at

Figure 3 The transverse arch of the hand. At the level of the MCP joints and also the PIP joints, the shape and depth of the arch changes with movements to open and close the hand.

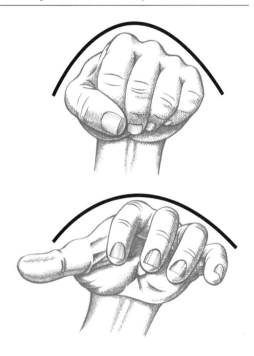

Figure 4 An X-ray of the wrist and hand. Note the normal longitudinal alignment of the bones in the forearm and hand.

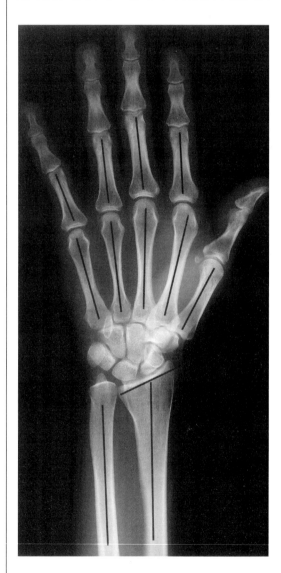

the carpal and metacarpal levels, whilst the longitudinal arches for each finger are formed by the carpals, metacarpal and the mobile phalanges. The depth of the transverse arch at the heads of the metacarpals, and the orientations of the longitudinal arches the ring and little fingers, change owing to the mobility of the fourth and fifth metacarpals at the carpometacarpal (CMC) joints, thus orientating the fingers to the thumb with increasing flexion. With flexion of the ring and little fingers, the heads of the finger metacarpals form an oblique angle to the transverse plane of the forearm. Oblique arches are formed between the thumb and each finger.

The longitudinal axis of the third metacarpal and radius align at rest, with some degrees of deviation at other metacarpals (Figure 4). Deviation of the proximal phalanges on the metacarpals is evident in ulnar deviation in the index, middle and little fingers. The progressive decrease in length of the finger metacarpals means the metacarpophalangeal (MCP) joints together form an oblique angle to the longitudinal axis of the forearm.

The dynamic structures of the hand, i.e. the transverse, longitudinal and oblique arches, are associated with the two oblique angles created by the changing length and mobility of the finger metacarpals. Thus, joint architecture must be respected in both design and fabrication of any wrist splint. Splints are generally higher and longer on the radial side.

Muscle Function

With the exception of flexor carpi ulnaris, which has fibres inserting on the pisiform and triquetrum, all wrist muscles insert directly on to the metacarpals. The arrangement of extrinsic finger and thumb muscles, and wrist muscles around the axis of wrist motion provides an agonist antagonist system of forces. Whilst effecting joint motion, the wrist musculature also provides significant stability. The position of the wrist has implications for the function of the thumb and fingers. The finger flexor muscles are lengthened as the wrist is extended, thus increasing their potential to generate force in grip. Similarly, the finger extensors are lengthened as they cross the greater arc of the flexed wrist, thus passively extending the fingers. The position of the thumb in relation to the fingers is also influenced by the degree of wrist flexion. Wrist extension is a more important motion than flexion owing to its association with finger flexion and the fact that many functional tasks require antigravity action of the wrist. Thus, functional splints tend to require positions of wrist extension. Substitution of wrist extensor action can be achieved by splinting.

Limitations in the excursion of the muscle tendon units that cross the wrist will dictate the positions the distal joints assume as the wrist position is changed. Limited excursion in the flexor digitorum superficialis and profundus will compromise finger and wrist extension. Finger extension is possible with significant degrees of wrist flexion; however, increasing finger flexion is seen with greater degrees of wrist extension. Similarly tightness in extensor digitorum will limit composite flexion of digital joints. The degrees of wrist extension will determine the total digital flexion possible. Passive motion of individual joints can be normal.

Extrinsic finger muscles arise in the proximal forearm with long tendons secured by retinaculum on the dorsal aspect of the wrist, and the retinaculum and carpal tunnel on the volar aspect of the wrist. Inflammation in these regions can affect the glide and function of the tendons with potential to compromise the median nerve in the carpal tunnel. Splinting is commonly used to limit tendon glide through the retinaculum to facilitate resolution of inflammation.

Soft Tissue Covering to the Wrist and Hand

Any splints applied to the wrist and hand must consider the skin and fascial coverings in the areas they traverse. The ability of tissues to withstand pressure has implications to the design.

The skin on the palm of the hand is quite different to that covering the dorsum of the hand and forearm. It has little mobility and is designed to withstand the pressure and shear characteristic of functional grip and pinch. Palmar skin is thick and firmly adhered to the underlying palmar aponeurosis by numerous fibrous connections.

Palmar blood vessels and nerves run deep to these structures prior to branching to run medially and laterally to each finger.

Dorsal skin is thin and very mobile. Only a thin subcutaneous sheet of fascia is located superficial to the extensor tendons over the metacarpals. The superficial venous system is visible. Application of pressure to the volar surface of the hand is not associated with the same risks as that to the dorsum of the hand. Here the skin, and venous and lymphatic drainage can be compromised as there is little fascia to disperse pressure being applied through these structures to the underlying bony surface. Bony prominences elsewhere in the hand and wrist present similar risks.

Skin creases are used as a guide to underlying structures for splint boundaries. As seen in Figure 5, the location of skin creases does not directly correlate to the underlying joints.

Figure 5   The skin creases of the hand. The skin creases are lines of tethering of the skin and, therefore, do not bear a direct relationship to the underlying joint.

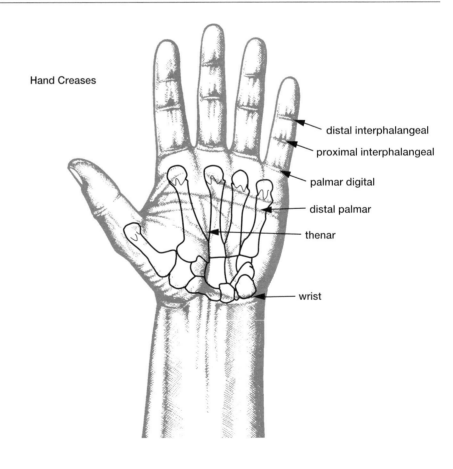

Hand Creases

distal interphalangeal

proximal interphalangeal

palmar digital

distal palmar

thenar

wrist

Splints Designed to Immobilize the Wrist and Hand

Immobilization of the wrist is undertaken to allow the wrist and associated tissues to rest in a position that minimizes complications associated with inflammation, contracture or paralysis. Immobilizing the wrist, but allowing movement in the fingers and thumb, may facilitate greater functional use of the hand.

Immobilization for Rest

At normal physiological rest, the wrist, thumb and fingers adopt a posture that represents a balance of muscular and ligamentous tension in the hand. A resting splint aims to restore this balance in the presence of trauma or disease. The resting position, common to the majority of persons, is 10°–20° wrist extension, 20°–45° flexion of the finger MCP joints, and between 10° and 30° flexion of the finger interphalangeal (IP) joints. The functional position assumed by joints of the hand may vary widely depending upon the vocational, avocational and self-care tasks undertaken at any point in time. Therefore, adopting one 'functional position' to rest the hand is inappropriate.

Although it may seem a statement of the obvious, a resting splint should position the hand in a *resting* position and not a *functional* position. However, on occasions, a position close to function may be chosen for immobilization at rest because this position offers the best functional outcome should mobility not be restored.

WRIST AND HAND IMMOBILIZATION SPLINTS

Immobilization of the hand and wrist is achieved with a splint applied to the volar surface addres-

Figure 6 Wrist hand immobilization splint. Support for inflamed or painful joints is achieved by a splint worn during non-functional periods of rest and sleep. Straps are positioned to avoid bony prominences.

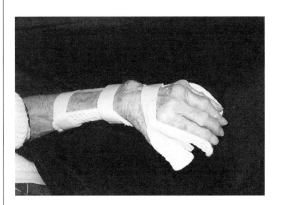

sing the wrist, fingers and thumb (Figure 6). It is indicated in the presence of paralysis, pain, inflammation and infection. If used in the presence of spasticity of the wrist and finger musculature, greater attention must be paid to design and location of straps, as these apply significant force to sustain the hand in the splint. An alternative wrist immobilization splint for use with clients with spasticity is discussed in Chapter 8. The splint position is determined by the pathology of the tissues with specific moulding to achieve a safe position of immobilization in those cases at risk of contracture. Figure 7 illustrates a splint design for situations where the thumb CMC and MCP joints are very painful or unstable, and require additional support on the volar surface.

Procedure to take a pattern Lay the plastic pattern material on a flat surface and place the patient's hand on top. The wrist should be between neutral and 10° ulnar deviation, the thumb comfortably extended with the fingers very slightly abducted.

Figure 7   Resting splint for the wrist and hand with palmar thumb support. Moulding this splint requires particular attention to the thumb position to ensure it is supported on the anterior surface in a resting position of slight CMC abduction and extension.

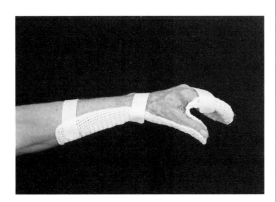

The length of the splint from wrist to proximal end is generally two-thirds the length of the forearm. This roughly equates to the length of the hand. Measure the length using a tape measure and mark it with a small dot.

Mark the following points on the pattern referring to Figure 8a.

1–2   Medial and lateral aspects of the hand just proximal to the heads of the finger metacarpals.

3–4   Medial and lateral aspects of the wrist at mid-carpal level.

5–6   Medial and lateral aspects of the forearm at length previously determined.

7   Tip of the middle finger.

8   The index and middle finger web.

The width of the splint should be half the circumference at the wrist and forearm, and slightly wider at the finger MCP joints so that the material will support the sides of the index and little fingers. This can be determined by wrapping the pattern material around the hand and marking the desired width at the forearm, wrist and finger MCPs. These width points are indicated on Figure 8b as la, 2a, 4a, etc.

Remove the patient's hand. Figure 8b is a volar view of the hand and illustrates how the pattern accommodates the specific land marks. To follow this diagram, work on the wrong side of the material used to take the pattern.

To shape the pattern:

1. Join points 1 and 2 (MCP line).
2. Join points 3 and 4 (wrist line).
3. Draw a vertical line from point 7 to intersect the wrist line.
4. Draw a vertical line from point 8 to intersect the MCP line — point 9. These lines are used as a guide to determine the location of the thenar crease.
5. Starting at point 7 draw a line around the fingers through points 2a, 4a and 6a, curve sharply around to 5a then up to 3. The curve through 5a should be shallow to ensure this aspect of the splint does not impede elbow flexion.
6. Draw a line between 3 and 9 following the thenar crease so it touches the vertical line from 7 approximately one-third of the distance between the wrist line and the MCP line, then curve to point 9.
7. From point 3, draw around the base of the thenar eminence to connect to la following on to point 7.
8. Cut the pattern out and check for fit on the patient prior to transferring it to the thermoplastic material.

Fabrication procedure

1. The arm should be positioned with the elbow supported, the forearm in a vertical position in mid-pronation–supination and the wrist in the

Figure 8 Pattern for a wrist hand immobilization splint. Landmarks are recorded as shown in (a) with the completed pattern applied to the volar surface of application (b).

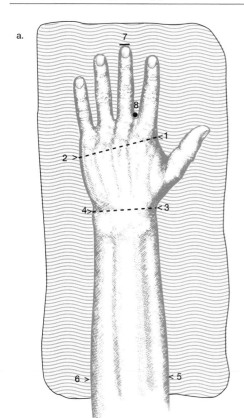
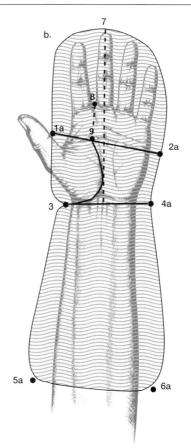

predetermined position, and the rest of the hand relaxed.

2. Heat the splinting material and cut out the pattern shape. Reheat.

3. On removing the material from the heating source, quickly shape the thumb component, particularly the index thumb webspace, using your own hand as a mould.

4. Place the splinting material on the patient's hand, orientating the alignment at the MCP joint and wrist. Where necessary, secure material to the wrist, hand and then forearm using a smooth bandage.

5. When splinting patients with a flail wrist, e.g. persons with quadriplegia, a second person may be required to assist bandaging the splinting material to the limb. If no assistance is available, bandage the material to the limb at the wrist first, then loosely bandage around the hand and fingers before sweeping back to secure the forearm component.

6. Now hold the wrist and finger joints in the desired position, while moulding the transverse and longitudinal arches. The thumb component may be moulded at a second stage, if it

is not possible to address all components in the first application.

7. When satisfied with the position of the hand in the splint, a minimum of three straps are applied. Straps are located at the proximal end, in the vicinity of the wrist, and either across the metacarpals or the proximal phalanges.

WRIST IMMOBILIZATION SPLINT (VOLAR THUMB DESIGN)

To design a wrist immobilization splint that provides support to the volar surface of the thumb the pattern is modified slightly as illustrated in Figure 9. An additional marker is added at the end of the thumb. The fabrication procedure is the same as that described for the wrist immobilization splint.

Immobilization for Function

Splints that immobilize the wrist without involvement of the fingers and thumb may be applied to rest the wrist but generally facilitate functional use of the hand. The angle of immobilization of the wrist is determined in consultation with the

Figure 9 Pattern for a wrist hand immobilization splint with an anterior thumb component. Landmarks are recorded as shown in (a) with the completed pattern applied to the volar surface of application (b).

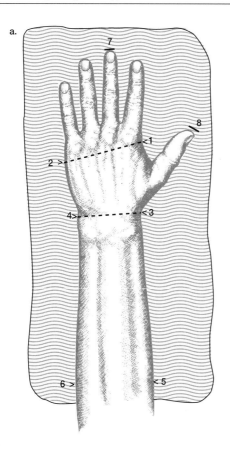
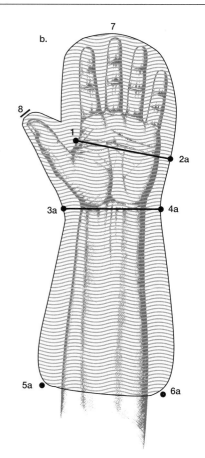

patient considering their specific requirements in occupational tasks. Research by Stewart and Mass (1990) suggests that no wrist splint design fulfils all functional criteria with certain splints better suited to specific patient characteristics and functional tasks than others.

Following assessment and determination of an objective for immobilization of the wrist, the therapist must consider the choices in the design, taking into consideration the pathology and the specific needs of the patient. The design choices are:

- **Volar splints** support the weight of the hand against the effect of gravity. The palmar skin is well able to tolerate pressure applied by the splint. Volar splints are designed for primary function in a pronated position. Aesthetically, the majority of splinting is located on the volar surface with only straps traversing the more exposed dorsal surface. The major disadvantage to this type of splint is the presence of hard unyielding plastic in the palm of the hand. This has the potential to compromise gross grip by preventing adaptation of the hand to the shape of the object.

- **Dorsal splints** are used for a small population of patients who require wrist support but with greater palmar surface exposed for sensory and friction contact with objects. Perhaps the least supportive of the wrist splint designs, dorsal wrist splints are popular with persons with rheumatoid arthritis who require support but rarely transmit large forces through their wrists.

- **Circumferential splints** provide the greatest amount of immobilization and support. Owing to their inherent strength in design, they are used in vocational situations where large forces are transmitted through the wrist. This design also provides uniform pressure dispersion

along the forearm and is, therefore, used in young children who still have considerable subcutaneous fat, and for those patients with significant swelling in the hand and forearm, which may be compromised by straps.

The use of prefabricated splints to immobilize the wrist may be an appropriate first aid intervention. However, the elastic nature of the fabric of most of these splints suggests their primary function is to restrict motion and not to immobilize the joint.

VOLAR WRIST IMMOBILIZATION SPLINT

This is perhaps the most traditional design for wrist immobilization splints (Figure 10). It requires a material that is strong and rigid as the component through the wrist is quite narrow. This splint is designed to be used in a pronated position and, therefore, should never be moulded to the hand with the forearm in supination. Splinting materials that require a gravity-assisted moulding technique are not recommended.

Procedure to take a pattern Lay the pattern material on a flat surface and place the patient's hand on the top. The wrist should be between

Figure 10 Volar wrist immobilization splint. This splint immobilizes the wrist in the required degrees of extension without effecting motion of the fingers and thumb.

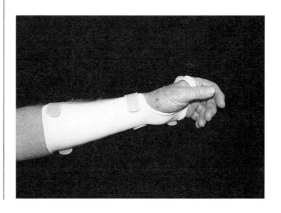

neutral and 10° ulnar deviation, the thumb comfortably extended, with the fingers very slightly abducted. The length of the splint from wrist to proximal end is generally two-thirds of the length of the forearm. This roughly equates to the length of the hand. Measure the length using a tape and mark it with a small dot.

Mark the following points as illustrated in Figure 11a.

1–2 Medial and lateral aspects of the hand just proximal to the heads of the finger metacarpals.

3–4 Medial and lateral aspects of the wrist at mid-carpal level.

5–6 Medial and lateral aspects of the forearm at the length previously determined.

7 The tip of the middle finger.

8 The index and middle finger web.

The width of the splint should be half the circumference at the wrist and forearm, and to the dorsal aspect of the fifth metacarpal. This can be determined by wrapping the pattern material around and marking the desired width at the MCP, fore-

Figure 11 Pattern for a volar wrist immobilization splint. Landmarks are recorded as shown in (a) with the completed pattern applied to the volar surface of application (b). Extra length is added to the distal edge as indicated by the dotted line.

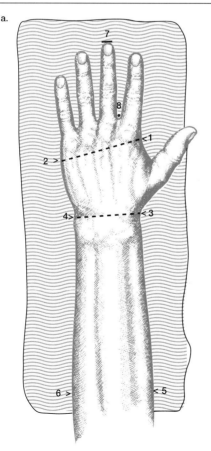

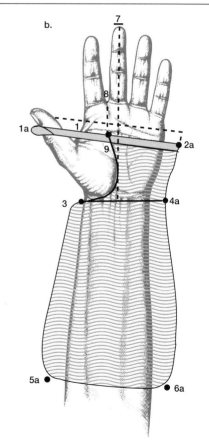

arm and wrist. These width points are indicated on the diagram as 2a, 4a, etc.

The distal end of this splint is extended to wrap around the hand through the web space. Using a tape, measure the width from the dorsum of the little finger metacarpal head across the volar aspect of the finger MCP joints, through the webspace to the dorsum of the middle finger metacarpal. This length is used to determine width of the distal end of the splint (1a–2a).

Remove the patient's hand. Figure 1lb is a volar view of the hand and how the pattern accommodates the specific land marks. To follow this diagram, work on the wrong side of the material used to take the pattern.

1. Join points 1 and 2 (MCP line).
2. Join points 3 and 4 (wrist line).
3. Draw a vertical line from point 7 to intersect the wrist line.
4. Draw a vertical line from point 8 to intersect the MCP line – point 9. These lines are used as a guide to determine the location of the thenar crease.
5. Starting at point 2a, draw a line around the forearm through points 4a and 6a, curve sharply around to 5a then up to 3. The curve through 5a should be shallow to ensure this aspect of the splint does not impede elbow flexion.
6. The line between 3 and 9 follows the thenar crease and so touches the vertical line 7 approximately one-third of the distance between the wrist line, and the MCP line then curves to point 9.
7. Extend the palmar bar using circumferential measurement previously recorded (1a–2a).
8. Add approximately 1 cm across the palmar surface distal to the MCP line. The additional length, indicated by a dotted line, allows the distal end to be rolled back to create a smooth edge.
9. Cut the pattern out and check for fit on the patient, ensuring the forearm is maintained in mid-prone or a pronated position. Transfer the pattern to the thermoplastic material.

Fabrication procedure
1. The arm should be positioned with the elbow supported, the forearm in a vertical position in mid-pronation–supination and the wrist in the predetermined position. Allow room for the changing dimensions of the distal ulna by padding out the ulna head prior to fabrication.
2. Heat the splinting material and cut out the pattern.
3. Fold back the component added distal to 1a and 2a to the level of the MCP line, with the exception of the last 2 cm at 1a. This section will provide a flat surface for the attachment of a strap. Ensure that the fold is towards the exterior surface of the splint as the rolled edge decreases shear stress and improves comfort whilst also providing reinforcement.
4. Reheat the material until malleable, then apply it to the patient's hand and secure it in place with a bandage. Mould it intimately around the wrist, the thenar eminence and the arches of the hand. Flare it around the edge of the thenar eminence and the proximal edge of the forearm.
5. Attach three straps, one at the proximal end, one in the vicinity of the wrist avoiding direct pressure over the ulna head and one to the bar at the distal end.
6. Ensure correct fit and that movement of the fingers at the MCP joints and the CMC joint of the thumb is not compromised.

DORSAL WRIST IMMOBILIZATION SPLINT

This splint requires a material that is strong and rigid. As the splint is designed to be used in a pronated position, gravity-assisted splinting materials can be used. These materials are also recommended owing to their ability to contour very well to the hand. The ulna head is padded out prior to fabrication.

Figure 12   Dorsal wrist immobilization splint. This splint meets the patient's functional requirements for wrist support (a) while maximizing the palmar surface available to contact the bowl (b).

---

a

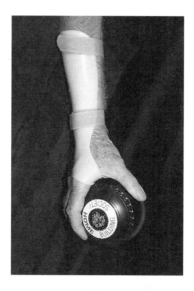

b

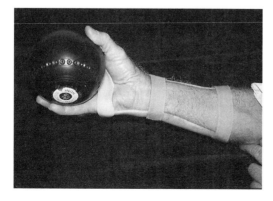

To support the transverse arch, a rigid splinting component must be incorporated into the design to traverse the palm of the hand proximal to the distal palmar crease. A flexible strap provides no support for the transverse arch. The first pattern described here has an extension on the radial side, which wraps through the webspace across the palm. This style is recommended for dorsal splints whose purpose is to facilitate function. A more supportive hinged palmar component is added to this splint design when it is used as a basis for dynamic splints or where greater palmar support is required.

Procedure to take a pattern

1. Lay the patient's hand on a flat surface and place the transparent plastic pattern material on top. The wrist should be between neutral and 10° ulnar deviation, with the thumb comfortably extended and the fingers very slightly abducted.
2. The length of the splint from the wrist to the proximal end is two-thirds of the length of the forearm. This roughly equates to the length of the hand. Measure the length using a tape and mark it with a small dot.

The following points, illustrated in Figure 13a, are common to all models:

1–2   Medial and lateral aspects of the hand just proximal to the heads of the finger metacarpals.

3–4   Medial and lateral aspects of the hand at the thumb web level.

5–6   Medial and lateral aspects of the wrist at mid-carpal level.

7–8   Medial and lateral aspects of the forearm at the length previously determined.

9   The index and middle finger web.

Figure 13   Pattern for a dorsal wrist immobilization splint. Landmarks are recorded as shown in (a) with the completed pattern applied to the dorsal surface of application (b). The narrow palmar bar is an extension of the dorsal pattern. The pattern for an extended palmar bar is illustrated in (c).

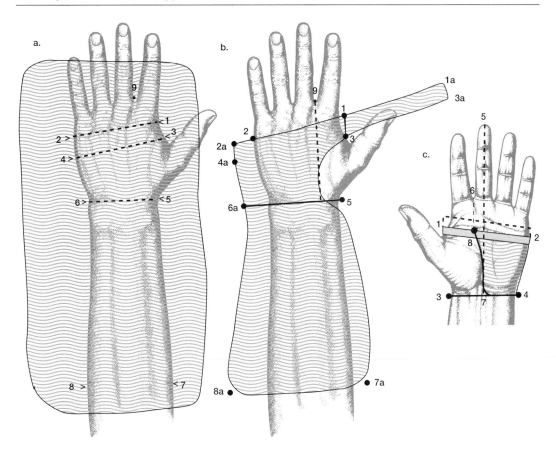

The width of the splint should be half the circumference of the forearm and wrist, and support the ulnar aspect of the fifth metacarpal. Wrap the pattern material around the hand and mark the desired width at the fifth MCP joint, forearm and wrist. Width points are indicated on the diagram as 2a, 4a, etc.

Remove the patient's hand and shape the pattern (Figure 13b).

1. Join points 1 and 2 (MCP line).
2. Join points 3 and 4 (thumb line).
3. Join points 5 and 6 (wrist line).

4. Draw a vertical line from point 9 to intersect the wrist line.
5. Starting at point 2a, draw a line around the forearm through points 4a, 6a and 8a, curve sharply around to 7a then up to 5. The curve through 7a should be shallow to ensure this aspect of the splint does not impede elbow flexion.
6. The line between 5 and 3 touches the vertical line 9 allowing clearance for the extensor pollicus longus (EPL) tendon during thumb extension.
7. To incorporate the palmar bar into the dorsal

97

pattern, the distal end of the splint is extended through the web space, across the palm of the hand to overlap slightly on the ulnar side of the splint. Using a tape, measure the circumference of finger metacarpals just proximal to the MCPs. Extend the MCP and thumb web lines according to the MCP circumferential measurement (2–1a).

8. Cut the pattern out and check for fit on the patient prior to transferring it to the thermoplastic material.

Fabrication procedure

1. The arm should be positioned with the elbow supported, the forearm in a vertical position in mid-pronation–supination and the wrist in the predetermined position. Allow room for the changing dimensions of the distal ulna by padding out the ulna head prior to fabrication.

2. Remove the thermoplastic material from the heating source. Gently flare the distal component from 1 to 1a to decrease shear stress and improve comfort.

3. Apply to the patient's hand and secure in place with a bandage. Mould intimately around the wrist, the arches of the hand, and gently flare the proximal and distal ends.

4. Attach three straps, one at the proximal end, one in the vicinity of the wrist and one to the bar at the distal end.

To extend the palmar component, to give greater support to the palmar aspect of the hand, an additional component can be made or incorporated into the dorsal pattern (Figure 14).

Mark the following points as illustrated in Figure 13c:

1–2 Medial and lateral aspects of the hand just proximal to the heads of the finger metacarpals.

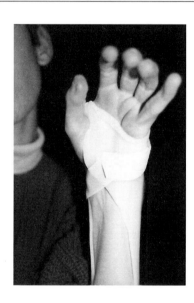

Figure 14 Dorsal wrist immobilization splint with an extended palmar bar. The palmar component may be incorporated into the dorsal pattern as illustrated or hinged in place with straps. The palmar component of this splint has been extended to achieve some abduction of the thumb.

3–4 Medial and lateral aspects of the wrist at radiocarpal level.

5　　The tip of the middle finger.

6　　The index and middle finger web.

To shape the pattern:

1. Join points 1 and 2 (MCP line).

2. Join points 3 and 4 (wrist line).

3. Draw a vertical line from point 5 to intersect the wrist line – point 7.

4. Draw a vertical line from point 6 to intersect the MCP line – point 8. These lines are used as a guide to determine the location of the thenar crease.

5. Draw a line from 2 to 4, then across the wrist to point 7.

6. The line between 7 and 8 follows the thenar crease.

This component is cut and moulded to the hand with the dorsal splint in place. Straps are used to secure it on ulnar and radial aspects. One set of straps can be attached permanently.

CIRCUMFERENTIAL WRIST IMMOBILIZATION SPLINT

This splint uses the principle of contour to provide rigidity (Figure 15), therefore, thick rigid splinting material is unsuitable. Climatic and vocational demands will determine the type of material, its thickness and, in the case of thermoplastic materials, the degree of perforation. Orfit®Classic or Orfit®Soft 1.6 mm or 2 mm thickness is the preferred thermoplastic splinting material for this type of wrist splint. Orfit®Soft is recommended for the novice therapist as the coating makes it easier to handle.

The preference of the author is for the opening to be located along the dorsal aspect of the hand. This ensures there is a complete, well-contoured rigid palmar bar for support, and that radial and ulnar deviation are well controlled. Location of the opening along the ulnar border of the hand allows

Figure 15 Circumferential wrist immobilization splint. The dorsal opening of this circumferential wrist splint ensures that the transverse arch is completely supported, and no radial or ulnar deviation can occur. Finger and thumb motion is not restricted in performance of occupational tasks.

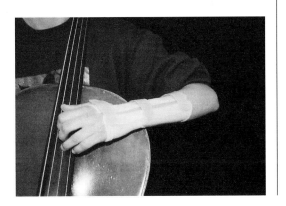

for easier access; however, palmar and ulnar support is less rigid owing to the strap location.

Orfit® material is available in precut patterns in three sizes with the opening located on the ulnar side. The following guide is provided for therapists to make their own patterns. Measurements for this splint pattern are all taken with a tape measure (see Figure 16).

Procedure to take a pattern For a dorsal opening, the hole for the thumb is located two-thirds from one edge of the material.

1–2 (and 3a–4a) Circumference around the heads of the finger MCP joints.

1–3a (and 2–4a) Length of the splint.

1–5 Two-thirds the MCP circumference.

5–2 One-third the MCP circumference.

1–1a and 2–2a The difference in length of the index compared to the little finger metacarpal. Approximately 1–1.5 cm in adults.

5–6 The length from the head of the index finger metacarpal to the head of the thumb metacarpal with the thumb in an adducted position. Approximately 2 cm in adults.

3–4 Circumference of the forearm.

3–3a and 4–4a The difference between the MCP and forearm circumference. This is divided evenly each side.

The hole for the thumb is located in the middle of the piece of splinting material when the opening is on the ulnar side.

1–2 The MCP circumference.

5–2 Half the MCP circumference.

When using materials without coating, cover any wound dressings with a thin layer of gauze to prevent removal of the dressing when removing

Figure 16   Pattern for a circumferential wrist immobilization splint. The pattern dimensions are determined by the circumferential and length measurements.

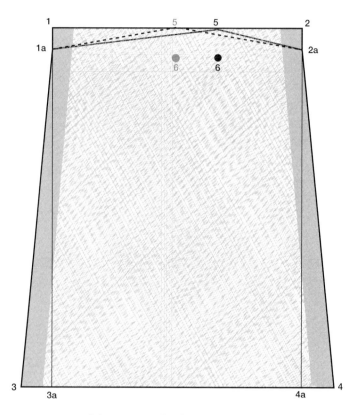

- - - - - - - - - Relate to pattern for ulnar opening

the splinting material from the arm. Remove non-stick coating along the length of the splint join (shaded in Figure 16) prior to heating materials with coating.

Fabrication procedure

1. Position the limb in a vertical position and determine the degree of extension required at the wrist. Ensure that the thumb is in a position of opposition.
2. Remove the material from the water by the distal ends. Enlarge the hole slightly and place the patient's thumb through it.
3. Wrap the material around the hand and press the distal edges together on the dorsum of the metacarpals.
4. Wrap the proximal ends around the forearm and press together on the dorsum of the forearm. Now the proximal and distal ends are secured, so your hands are free to mould the rest of the splint.
5. Join the two edges along the length of the splint, ensuring excess material is taken towards the seam on the dorsal surface.
6. Forceful moulding is not required with this

material; however, it is necessary to contour around the wrist and palmar arches.

7. When the material is cool but before it goes completely hard, separate the bond and carefully remove the splint from the patient's hand.

8. If the seam on the opening is not of even width along the length of the splint, the excess is trimmed.

9. Reheat the seam width. Then turn it down on the splint to provide reinforcement.

10. The distal end is also rolled back to provide a rounded edge allowing full motion at the MCP joints. Similarly, the proximal end is heated and folded back on itself.

11. If thumb motion is allowed, the thumb component is heated and a slightly larger hole cut. The edges are rolled back to allow freedom of motion of the thenar muscles. The component in the webspace between the thumb and index finger must have a smooth round edge to minimize problems of friction.

12. Three straps are then applied to secure the splint.

Wrist splint with thumb component If the pathology requires both the wrist and the thumb to be immobilized, an additional component may be added to this splint (Figure 17). To achieve this, all of the above stages, with the exception of step 11, are completed including application of straps. A small piece of thermoplastic splinting material is then added. It is slightly larger than the length and circumference of the proximal phalanx and overlaps the splint to bond approximately 1 cm.

The heated material is positioned around the thumb and the seam cut whilst warm. Prior to the material going hard, the circumference around the proximal phalanx is enlarged slightly to allow for the greater diameter of the IP joint.

Figure 17 Immobilization of the thumb MCP joint is achieved by the addition of an extra piece of material.

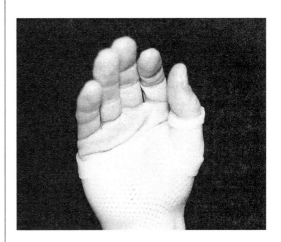

The heat-sealed seam is then reinforced with an additional piece of material. The distal end is rolled to allow full IP joint motion.

Splints Designed to Mobilize the Wrist

Mobilization splints fabricated for the wrist either address deficits in passive range of motion (ROM) of the wrist and extrinsic finger muscles, or redirect muscle action to facilitate motion in the presence of paralysis. Splinting techniques used to mobilize the wrist in the presence of spasticity are discussed in Chapter 8.

Splints to Address Deficits in Passive ROM in the Wrist

The requirements for joint motion vary according to the patient's functional and vocational activities. Numerous studies have been undertaken with various types of measuring devices; however, the findings are not dissimilar to those of Ryu *et al.* (1991). Extension-orientated ranges of motion were seen accompanying daily living activities requiring continuous movement. Perineal care required the greatest amounts of wrist flexion.

Mobilizing wrist splints apply force to both the radiocarpal and mid-carpal joints. Here, application of force perpendicular to the longitudinal axis of the second and third metacarpals is essential to avoid translational force compressing the joints. Serial progressive and dynamic splints are recommended for adults, with static serial splints recommended for children. Experience suggests that the majority of patients can tolerate mobilizing splints through the first 40° in extension and flexion for periods of time up to 3 hours. However, tolerance time is generally not greater than 1 hour in ranges of motion greater than 40°.

Serial static splints use a volar wrist design to address deficits in extension, with the dorsal wrist design for deficits in flexion. These splints need to be totally remoulded as range changes. Although the cost is higher, serial static splints are generally used to resolve deficits in ROM in young children thus eliminating problems associated with getting appropriate size hinges and risks of using dynamic traction.

Serial progressive and dynamic wrist-mobilizing splints have forearm- and hand-based components connected by some form of hinge. This hinge prevents the migration of the splint components and deviation of the wrist. Alignment of the axis of the hinge to the axis of flexion/extension of the wrist is essential. Care is taken to ensure that alteration in the arc of motion subsequent to fracture and/or surgery is accommodated. Often the shape of the forearm, progressively getting smaller towards the wrist, makes stabilization of the forearm component

difficult unless it is anchored around the flexed elbow (see Figure 21). This becomes a greater issue on small or thin arms, or when force is being applied to the wrist with an angle greater than 40°. An elbow component is more cumbersome but is more comfortable as it minimizes shear stress. A circumferential arm component, with the opening located on the medial surface, is more comfortable as it disperses pressure well.

Serial progressive splints use hinges that can be changed to increase the passive range of motion (PROM) into flexion or extension (Figure 18). Commercial hinge designs, available for the wrist joint from major splinting material suppliers, have locking devices that can be changed with a small key. The joint is locked at the end of available PROM. As tissue responds the end range is gradually increased.

Hinges may be located on either the radial or the ulnar side of the wrist, and secured to the components moulded around the hand and forearm. It is necessary to try the hinge in both positions to ensure you use the one that best accommodates for the change in dimension from the forearm to the hand. To minimize wrist deviation, an additional layer of splinting material may be required in the area where the hinge is bonded to the hand or forearm components.

Serial progressive splints are cost effective in that only modification to the joint angle is necessary as ROM improves. Most patients can be taught to undertake this task.

Where cost and availability prohibit the use of hinges, dynamic splints are used with an articulating swivel joint at the wrist (Figures 19 and 20). The joint can be made from screw rivets.

The hand component must disperse pressure applied to mobilize the wrist, therefore, it should

Figure 18 Serial progressive wrist splint. A prefabricated hinge is used to sustain this wrist at the end range of flexion.

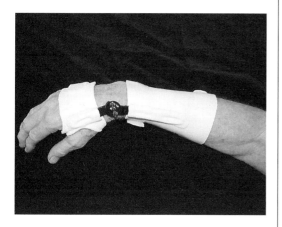

Figure 19 Dynamic wrist extension splint. This articulated splint prevents migration of components during force application. Long, strong elastic bands apply a mobilizing force at an angle determined by the outrigger.

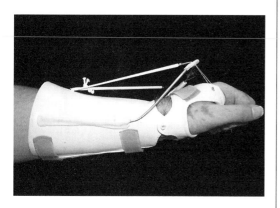

Figure 20 Dynamic wrist extension splint. The volar view illustrates the shape of the hand component. It allows movement of the fingers and thumb with extensions on the lateral aspect of the wrist to create the articulation. The design of the forearm component allows for attachment of an outrigger should there be a requirement to address wrist flexion.

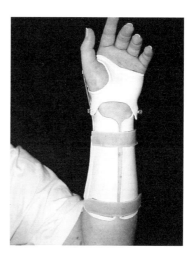

be well contoured and support all the finger metacarpals. In splints that address flexion, the pressure will be applied to the dorsal surface of the hand, therefore, the splinting material should disperse it over the length of the metacarpals. Ensure intimate contour and accommodate the transverse arch. Anchorage for pull is located on the volar surface. Extension force will be applied to the volar surface of the hand component. Therefore, it should have maximum contact with the palm of the hand without compromising motion of the fingers and thumb.

ARTICULATED WRIST SPLINT

Procedure for taking a pattern If a commercial hinge is to be used, first determine whether the hinge will be located on the radial or ulnar aspect of the wrist. The forearm component is circumferential as it ensures good contour and a large area for pressure dispersion, and minimizes potential rotation. The location of the opening is volar unless a flexion outrigger is to be used.

Take the following measurements with a tape measure:

1 Circumference of the wrist.
2 Circumference of the proximal forearm.
3 Length from the wrist to two-thirds the length of the forearm.

If this pattern is used for a dynamic splint with a swivel joint at the wrist, additional length is added to the medial and lateral aspects of the wrist. Fit it to the patient to ensure correct dimensions.

The pattern for the hand component, when using plastic rubber based splinting materials, is based upon the following measurements:

1　The width is equal to the circumference of the metacarpals.
2　The length is equal to the length of the index metacarpal from the distal palmar crease to the proximal wrist crease.
3　Punch a hole for the thumb. The location for this hole is determined by the location of the opening – one-third from one end in width and equidistant from the edges in length for either dorsal or volar openings, and in the centre for an ulnar opening.

Fabrication procedure
1.　Cut out forearm splinting material and heat.
2.　Apply the heated material, mindful of the location of the opening of the forearm component.
3.　Excess material on the volar and dorsal surfaces of the wrist is removed so that end range movement is not compromised. Additional length remains on the medial and lateral borders if a swivel hinge is to be used.
4.　Attach the Velcro® straps to the proximal and distal ends of the forearm component. If an outrigger is to be attached to address a flexion deficit just tape the splint together as the outrigger must be bonded to the splint prior to application of the straps.
5.　To secure the forearm component around the elbow, a wide Velcro® or Velfoam strap can be used. Alternatively, an additional piece of thermoplastic material is moulded around the back of the elbow positioned in approximately 90°

[Figure 21]. It is bonded to the medial and lateral aspects of the forearm component.
6.　Heat the hand splinting material, then roll back the edges of the hole to a size that will accommodate the thenar eminence.
7.　The thumb is placed through the hole and the material is moulded around the metacarpals and wrist. For a dynamic flexion splint, the join is placed on the volar surface. For a dynamic extension splint, the join is placed on the dorsal surface. When using a prefabricated hinge the opening is generally on the opposite side of the hand to the hinge. Good contour is essential.
8.　Ensure that movement of the MCP joints and thenar eminence has not been compromised. Excess material on the volar and dorsal surfaces of the wrist is removed so that end range movement is not compromised. Length on the medial and lateral borders allows for the swivel hinge.
9.　Attach the Velcro® strap.

The two components are then joined. The axis of the prefabricated hinge is aligned with the axis of the joint and location of the arms of the hinge marked on the hand and forearm components. The hinge is secured by an additional piece of splinting material. Splinting material can accommodate for the differences in contour between the hand component and the hinge, whereas the rivets supplied with the hinge can only be used where both the hinge and the splint surfaces are totally compatible. The joint is positioned at end range of passive motion and then the screws on the hinge secured.

For a dynamic splint where the mobilizing force is applied by dynamic traction, a swivel joint is necessary to prevent migration of components. To create a swivel joint, a hole slightly larger than the screw rivet is punched into the extensions on the hand component at the axis of joint motion on both radial and ulnar sides. Using the hole as a template, mark the location of the rivets on the small medial and lateral extensions of the forearm component. Secure the rivets by bonding it to the forearm component with a small piece of splinting material. This allows the hand piece to be removed from over the rivet to increase ease of access to the splint.

Complete the hand and forearm components and secure to the hand prior to determining the location of the outrigger and the dynamic traction. Traction is applied by elastic material to maintain the joint at end range, overcoming the effect of gravity and the weight of the hand. It is secured by small dress hooks melted into the thermoplastic on the radial and ulnar sides of the hand component.

One arm of the outrigger welding rod is shaped to contour the radial side of the forearm component. Then maintaining a low profile it is angled in the desired direction (flexion or extension). The radial side of the traction is applied perpendicular to the third metacarpal. The point of intersection of the traction with the welding rod determines the length of the outrigger. The outrigger is bent across the width of the hand, accommodating the ulnar side of the traction, prior to being angled along the ulnar side of the forearm component. The outrigger is secured to the forearm component by additional splinting material. A small piece of thermoplastic material is then moulded over the distal end of the outrigger with two holes created to maintain and direct the radial and ulnar traction. The eye of the dress hook is heated over the heat gun and positioned in the thermoplastic around the holes to minimize friction and prevent traction cutting through the splinting material. The traction is secured at the proximal end of the splint by a small dress hook melted into the thermoplastic. As range improves, modification to the alignment of the outrigger is undertaken by the therapist.

Splints to Address Deficits in Passive ROM in the Wrist and Fingers

Extrinsic flexor tendon unit tightness can modify the position of both the wrist and finger joints. This problem requires lengthy periods of splinting. To use a serial splint for this problem, the wrist is maintained between neutral and 20° flexion with the extending stress applied to the fingers (Figure 21). Only when the fingers can be extended with the wrist in neutral is extension of the wrist addressed. To address extrinsic flexor tendon tightness, the palmar side of the hand component is extended to include the whole volar surface of the fingers.

Figure 21 Dynamic wrist / finger splint. Where there is extrinsic flexor tendon tightness, a serial static component maintains a position for the fingers with the dynamic force directed to the wrist. An additional component is added to secure the splint around the elbow to prevent distal migration.

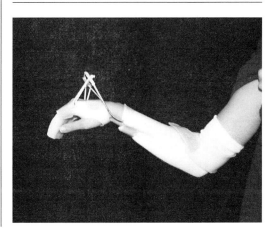

The technique for using serial plaster stretchers in the management of flexor tendon unit tightness is described by Tribuzi (1995). The principles follow those used in serial splinting. Indications for the use of plaster pertain to the cost, and the ability of the material to breathe and provide intimate contour.

Splinting to address extrinsic extensor tendon tightness requires a combination of wrist immobilization with a mobilizing force applied to the ends of the fingers. The focus is on gaining flexion of all finger joints, and techniques to achieve this are discussed in Chapter 6.

Wrist-mobilizing Splints – Paralysis and Spasticity

In the presence of paralysis, dynamic splints redirect active motion of non-paralysed muscles to effect motion in targeted joints. The unique coupling of the wrist and finger musculature in the tenodesis action allows a therapist to design splints to facilitate grip and pinch function. Where there is paralysis of finger flexor muscles, as is seen following a C6 spinal cord lesion, the action of the wrist extensors is harnessed to approximate fingers to the thumb for pinch. When there is paralysis of wrist and finger extensor muscles in radial nerve palsy, the reverse action is used with wrist flexion effecting finger extension.

The practice of using wrist-driven tenodesis splints, in acute management of persons with quadriplegia, varies between spinal rehabilitation units. The tenodesis orthosis is generally manufactured by orthotists. Patient-specific components are moulded from high-temperature thermoplastic materials thus requiring a positive–negative plaster mould. Whilst maximizing the potential for wrist movement to facilitate finger–thumb approximation for grip during table-based activities, the components cover a large proportion of the only sensate area of the hand and impede other functional tasks, such as wheelchair mobility and transfers. Continued use of these orthoses following discharge from hospital is quite low. Alternatively, judicious use of splinting to position the fingers in flexion to create shortening in the finger flexor tendons, combined with appropriate splinting to positioning the thumb in opposition, can result in an effective grasp and release in the long term. Whilst long-standing denervation can result in joint contractures, prior to addressing deficits in joint ROM, it should be determined that these contractures actually impede and do not facilitate hand function. Splints designed to augment and facilitate movement of the wrist in the presence of the wrist in the presence of spasticity are described in chapter 8.

PERIPHERAL NERVE SPLINTS

Of the peripheral nerve injuries affecting the wrist, the most common and the most significant, owing to the impact on function, is that affecting the radial nerve. Following injury to the radial nerve above the elbow, the characteristic deficit in wrist, finger and thumb extension is evident. The requirement is to position the wrist so that innervated flexor muscles can function effectively. Numerous splints are described which use combinations of immobilization of the wrist, with springs, elastic and non-elastic traction to mobilize the fingers. Crochetiere et al. (1975) first described a splint that used active flexor muscle function to substitute for the paralysed extensor musculature effectively without immobilization or need for springs (Figure 22). As the finger loops are attached directly to the outrigger, accuracy in

Figure 22   Radial nerve palsy splint. An outrigger secured to a long forearm base redirects wrist and finger action so that wrist extension is associated with active finger flexion (top) and finger MCP extension with active wrist flexion (bottom).

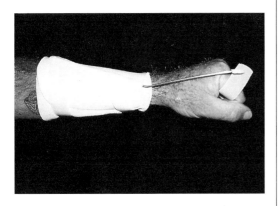

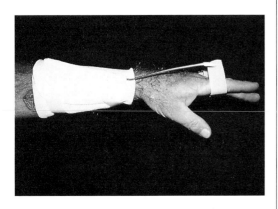

the alignment of the outrigger (Figure 24) is necessary for this splint to function effectively. This design was modified by Colditz (1987) to increase ease of fabrication for the therapist. A static line supports the finger loops, suspended by an outrigger that redirects the line of pull along the dorsum of the hand. Less precision is required in the manufacture of the outrigger with adjustment being in the lengths of the static lines for each finger. The author's experience with a design based upon the Granger orthosis suggest an easier manufacturing procedure.

The patient should gently grasp a cylindrical

shaped object so that the wrist is in 20°–30° extension, MCPs 45° flexion and the rest of the joints flexed. A rolled crepe bandage is good; however, a tool handle specific to the patient's trade is also appropriate. Take a piece of 3.2 mm brass welding rod 50 cm in length.

The outrigger traverses the lateral aspects of the forearm, is angled into extension at the wrist, then traverses across the middle of the proximal phalanges following the descending angle of the heads of the metacarpals. To bend the outrigger refer to Figure 23.

1–2   The length of the forearm component to the wrist, angle the rod at the wrist into 20°–30° extension.

2–3   From the wrist to the middle of the proximal phalanx allowing approximately 1 cm clearance to the top of the finger. This point is at 90° perpendicular to the middle of the proximal phalanx.

3–4   The width of the hand across the proximal phalanges plus 0.5 cm clearance on the medial and lateral sides. This component must also be angled to accommodate the decreasing lengths of the metacarpals. To accommodate the changing transverse arch of the hand, the metacarpal component is secured in a vice and then the finger component rotated medially.

4–5   1 cm distal to the top of the proximal phalanx of the little finger to the axis of the wrist.

5–6   The length of the forearm component.

Finger loops are measured with a tape measure allowing 1.5 cm above the dorsum of the finger on both sides. Holes are punched for insertion of the outrigger 0.5 cm from the edge. Finger loops are made from narrow Velcro® or very thin leather. If

Figure 23   Pattern for the outrigger of the radial nerve palsy splint. Thick brass welding rod is shaped according to the pattern illustrated. If extension abduction of the thumb is also required, the outrigger follows the broken line along the thumb metacarpal.

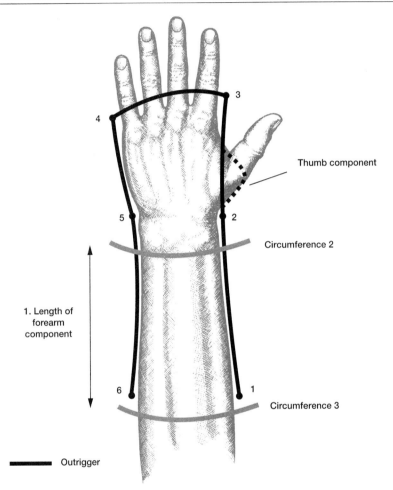

Thumb component

Circumference 2

1. Length of forearm component

Circumference 3

▬▬▬▬ Outrigger

the hand is to be used in water, Velcro® loops are recommended.

The pattern for the forearm component, to which the outrigger is attached, requires a series of length and circumferential measurements.

1 The length from just proximal to the ulna head to two-thirds the length of the forearm. Mark these two points to locate the next two circumferential measurements.
2 The circumference of the wrist just proximal to the ulna head.

3 The circumference of the proximal forearm.

Attach the finger loops to the outrigger and check the lengths prior to bonding the outrigger to the forearm component. Ensure alignment along the lateral aspects of the wrist and the hand. The bond should allow the outrigger to be pulled out so that the finger loop length may be adjusted and replaced when necessary. Attach the Velcro® straps at the proximal and distal ends of the forearm component.

This splint requires a period of supervised therapy

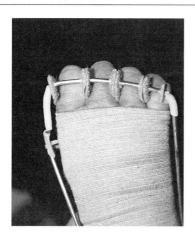

Figure 25   Radial nerve palsy splint. The alignment of the radial side of the outrigger is modified to facilitate thumb extension abduction.

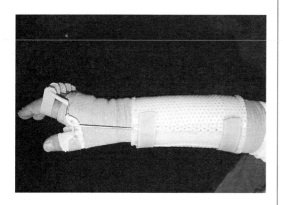

to ensure that the patient has an understanding of how to achieve efficient finger opening and closing. It is worn during the day to achieve functional goals with a splint to immobilize the wrist at night.

Many persons with radial nerve palsy can use abductor pollicus brevis to abduct the thumb sufficient for functional grip. However, if greater thumb extension is required, the outrigger is modified to follow the line of the thumb meta-carpal to the MCP joint with the thumb in slight extension. A loop around the thumb is attached to the outrigger with an elastic band so that extension is assisted when the wrist is flexed (Figure 25).

Splints Designed to Restrict Motion in the Wrist

Splints that restrict motion in the wrist are used for two groups of patients. The first group have sustained injuries to the carpals or distal radius and require limited movement to facilitate the healing of tissues. The second group are those persons with permanent disabilities, such as rheumatoid arthritis or cerebral palsy, where the wrist requires some form of support but not rigid immobilization. Recovery of, or sustaining functional movement of the wrist, is the primary objective of splinting for both groups. In selecting splints to restrict motion in the wrist, the therapist has a very large choice of prefabricated splints or the option to use customized splints.

Numerous designs are described in the literature that restrict wrist motion in either flexion extension, or radial and ulnar deviation. This is achieved by a hand and forearm component articulated by metal hinges or flexible thermoplastic tube (Bora *et al.*, 1989). These splints are manufactured using the hand and forearm components described in the previous section. Circumferential supports made from neoprene, cloth tape (Henshaw *et al.*, 1989) and silicone rubber (Canelón, 1995) are also used for early return to work or sport.

Prefabricated Elastic Wrist Splints

The prefabricated wrist splints have established a niche in the market owing to their accessibility in pharmacies and easy application by physicians and therapists. The hardness and rigidity of thermoplastic materials have often led to complications and diminished acceptance of these materials for fabrication of wrist splints. Materials that have greater drapability and contour, that are soft and light and do not rigidly immobilize a joint have proved to be more acceptable to persons with rheumatoid arthritis or other permanent disability. Kjeken *et al.* (1995), in a prospective study involving persons with inflammatory arthritis using an elasticized wrist splint over a 6-month period, found that pain was reduced and function improved. There was no evidence of a reduction in range of motion or grip strength as a consequence of wearing the splint.

A number of brands of prefabricated wrist splints, and many versions within each brand, regularly feature in advertisements in the therapy journals. The majority of these splints are made of elastic-based materials, reinforced on the volar surface with thermoplastic or metal, and secured by Velcro® tabs. The advantage of these splints is that they provide a significant saving in time and require no knowledge of splint fabrication. However, universal sizing to a 'normal-shaped' hand often results in inadequate support owing to poor fit, inadequate length, and impingement of motion of the thumb and MCP joints of the fingers (Henshaw *et al.* 1989) [Figure 26]. In addition, the difference in flexibility between the splint material and reinforcing bar will always allow movement between these two components, and between the hand and the splint. Taking the time to fit the appropriate size and modify reinforcing inserts to accommodate the shape of the patient's hand, are essential to ensure adequate support with restriction of motion limited to the wrist.

Figure 26   Commercially manufactured wrist splints. The smallest size prefabricated Futuro splint compromises both finger and thumb movement in the hand on the left. A second skin gauntlet splint on the right does not impede finger movement. Correct fit is an advantage of a customized splint.

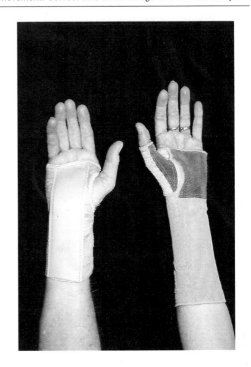

Custom-made Splints

Customized splints have advantages over prefabricated splints in accommodating the unique dimensions of the hand and the specific requirements of the pathology. Those persons who prefer a softer, more flexible splinting material or who have significant deformities require customized splints. Flexible materials used for customized splints can accommodate bony architecture but do not sustain any shape on concave surfaces. Therefore, contour can only be achieved by design, and by the manner in which components are sewn or held in place by reinforcement.

Commercially available custom-made splints have advantages over therapist-manufactured splints because of the expertise and equipment of the manufacturer. It allows for more choices in design, selection of materials and leads to a more professional finished product. Lycra® splints use directional lines of tension within several layers of Lycra® fabric to achieve the desired objective of assisting function of the wrist according to the patient's requirements. Measurement forms and prescription details are available from the manufacturer (Second Skin, 251 Adelaide Terrace, Perth, Western Australia 6000).

Less precise splints made of neoprene and Lycra® (Backman, 1988) are commonly manufactured by therapists using a domestic sewing machine. The 'bulk' of the neoprene and elasticity of Lycra® are used to restrict motion, with reinforcement added by pieces of thermoplastic materials. Components of reinforcement are determined by the stability required to address the forces transmitted through the hand.

NEOPRENE WRIST SPLINT PATTERN

The following pattern is detailed in relation to the thumb specifically to add contour to the carpal region. The pattern for this splint requires a series of circumferential and length measurements. Place the hand on a flat surface and mark the following points (Figure 27a and b):

1–2 The medial and lateral aspects of the hand just proximal to the heads of the finger metacarpals.

3 The thumb web just proximal to the MCP joint.

4–5 The medial and lateral aspects of the wrist at mid-carpal level.

6 Between the index and middle finger web.

7 The tip of the middle finger.

Mark a point at two-thirds of the length of the forearm.

Join points 1 and 2 (MCP line), and 4–5 (wrist line). Draw a line longitudinally through the finger from point 7 to intersect the wrist line. This line is the centre line of the pattern. Draw a vertical line from point 6 to intersect the MCP line.

Measure lengths using features identified in initial pattern (Figure 27c).

i   1–3 proximal to index MCP to base of thumb web just proximal to the thumb MCP joint volar surface.
ii   3 to thumb IP joint.
iii   Thumb MCP joint to the distal wrist crease.
iv   MCP line to wrist line at middle finger.
v   MCP line to wrist line ulnar side of the little finger.
vi   Wrist to the proximal end.

Measure the following circumferences using a tape:

1   Metacarpals at the level of the MCP line.

2   Wrist.

3–5   Circumferences of the forearm.

6   Thumb at IP joint.

7   Thumb just distal to the MCP joint.

Length and circumferential measurements are assembled into a final pattern as seen in Figure 27d. The thumb component is determined by the lengths between the IP and the MCP, and the MCP and the wrist. The distal width is two-thirds the circumference. The thumb component is sewn into the wrist component around the curve of the thenar eminence using a flat seam (join between 3 and 6a).

Figure 27   Pattern for a neoprene soft wrist splint. (a) An outline of the major landmarks of the hand. (b) The position of the thenar eminence in relation to the rest of the hand is determined using the points identified. (c) Length and circumferential measurements are indicated. (d) The pattern shape for the forearm component, the thumb and thumb gusset as determined by measurements.

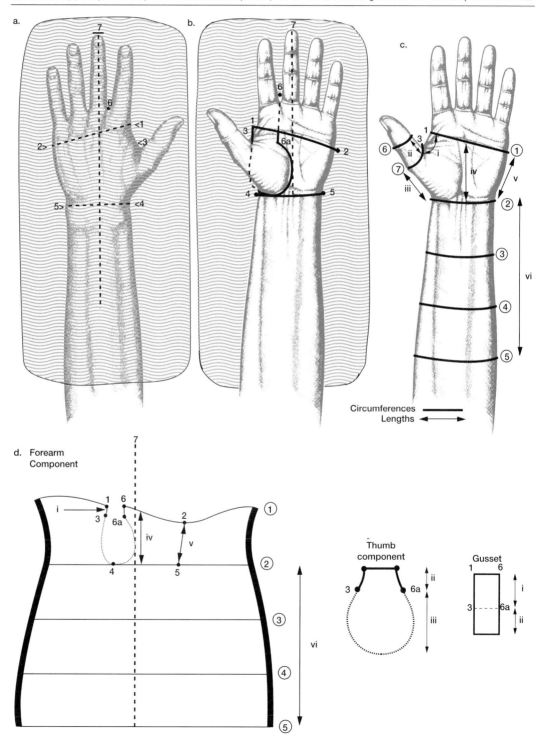

The gusset length is determined by adding the two thumb lengths through the webspace i and ii. The width of the gusset is one-third the circumference of the thumb. Match points 3 and 6a. The gusset is stitched to both the thumb component and the hand component.

Closing for this splint is achieved by Velcro® hook and pile attached to the length of the dorsal opening. However, insertion of a zipper provides a more convenient and effective fastening.

Conclusion

Wrist stability and mobility are critical factors in the successful use of the upper limb in a wide variety of functional and vocational activities. Subsequent to disease or injury affecting the wrist, these essential assets may be lost with significant consequences to function. Splinting is an extremely valuable therapeutic tool in the management of wrist dysfunction. Multiple designs and materials are used to immobilize, restrict or mobilize tissues according to the involved pathology and the occupational performance objectives of the patient.

References

Backman, C (1988) Spandex wrist splint: an alternative for the client with arthritis. *Canadian Journal of Occupational Therapy* **55**: 89–91.

Berger, RA (1996) The anatomy and basic biomechanics of the wrist joint. *Journal of Hand Therapy* **9**: 84–93.

Berger, RA, Garcia-Elias, M (1991) General anatomy of the wrist. In: An, K, Berger, R, Cooney, WP (eds) *Biomechanics of the Wrist Joint*, pp. 1–22. New York: Springer-Verlag.

Bora, FW, Culp, RW, Osterman, AL, Skirven T (1989) A flexible wrist splint. *Journal of Hand Surgery* **14A**: 574–575.

Canelón, MF (1995) Silicone rubber splinting for athletic hand and wrist injuries. *Journal of Hand Therapy* **8**: 252–257.

Colditz, JC (1987) Splinting for radial nerve palsy. *Journal of Hand Surgery* **1**: 18–23.

Crochetiere, W, Granger, CV, Ireland, J (1975) The 'Granger' orthosis for radial nerve palsy. *Orthotics and Prothetics* **27**: 27–31.

Henshaw, JL, Satren, JW, Wrightsman, JA (1989) The semi flexible wrist splint. *Journal of Hand Therapy* **2**: 35–40.

Kjeken, I, Møller, G, Kvien, TK (1995) Use of commercially produced elastic wrist orthoses in chronic arthritis: a controlled study. *Arthritis Care and Research* **8**: 108–113.

Palmer, AK (1988) Fractures of the distal radius. In: Green, DP (ed) *Operative Hand Surgery*, 2nd edn, pp. 991–1026. New York: Churchill Livingstone.

Ryu, J, Palmer, AK, Cooney, WP (1991) Wrist joint motion. In: An, KN, Berger, RA, Cooney, WP (eds) *Biomechanics of the Wrist Joint*, pp. 37–60. New York: Springer-Verlag.

Stewart, D, Mass, F (1990) Splint suitability: a comparison of four splints. *Australian Journal of Occupational Therapy* **37**: 15–24.

Tribuzi, S (1995) Serial plaster splinting. In: Hunter, JM, Makin, EJ, Callahan, AD (eds) *Rehabilitation of the Hand: Surgery and Therapy*, pp. 1599–1608. St Louis: Mosby.

Tubiana, R (1981) Architecture and functions of the hand. In: Tubiana, R (ed) *The Hand*, Vol. 1, pp. 19–93. WB Saunders: Philadelphia.

6

Splinting to Address the Fingers

Introduction

The fingers with their varying orientation and degrees of mobility provide the hand with an incredibly versatile tool to gain information through the sensory innervation of the skin and to transmit force in grasp and pinch. Stability and mobility of the fingers are required for the hand to achieve its unique functional requirements.

Fingers are vulnerable to injury and to the effects of diseases of the musculoskeletal system. Whilst often considered relatively minor, injuries to a finger can impact upon the whole hand and, therefore, functional performance of the individual. Splinting is used to provide joint stability and

protection of injured or repaired structures; however, in the majority of cases, it is used to restore mobility. This chapter will describe a variety of splints that are used to maximize functional potential of diseased or injured fingers.

Anatomy

Successful application of splints to the hand demands a sound knowledge of anatomy and kinesiology. The unique arrangements of the structural components of finger bones and joints, combined with the interconnections between intrinsic and extrinsic musculature, allow adapta-

Figure 1   The digital articular chain. It is designed to function in flexion. Each articulation has strong collateral ligaments and a volar plate. Reproduced from Tubiana (1981, p. 191).

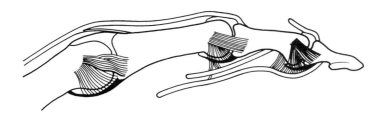

tion of shape with variance in force transmission for the many demands normal function requires.

The articulations of the fingers are designed to function in the direction of flexion. The capsule is reinforced with strong collateral ligaments, a volar plate and tendons that traverse the joints (Figure 1). The MCP joints are ball and socket joints allowing active motion in flexion and extension, abduction and adduction, and passive rotation. The shapes of the metacarpal heads, combined with slightly longer radial, as compared to ulnar, collateral ligaments, allows rotational motion during flexion.

The orientation of the longitudinal axis of the fingers varies from extension to flexion. Fess (1989) determined that convergence of this axis changed from an area at the base of the thumb for individual finger flexion to the radial distal half of the forearm in simultaneous flexion of all fingers (Figure 2). Variation between the orientation of the finger axis in extension as compared to flexion was greater in the index and little fingers. The wrist position did not influence convergence. Thus care is required to orientate the direction of force correctly in traction used to mobilize a finger, or fingers, into flexion.

The anatomical arrangement of the capsular structures of the MCP joints determines the safe position for immobilization. The collateral ligaments are located eccentrically with respect to the centre of rotation of the joint. Thus, the distance from origin to insertion of the collateral ligaments progressively increases during joint flexion reaching a plateau after 45° (Minami et al., 1985). Immobilizing MCP joints in 70°–90° flexion to maintain length in the collateral ligaments is a long-standing splinting practice (Fess and Philips, 1987; Boscheinen–Morrin et al., 1992). However, the study by Minami et al. (1985) would suggest a position greater than 45° of flexion will maintain length in the collateral ligaments of MCP joints. The tension of the ligaments in MCP flexion will restrict abduction movements at these joints.

The IP joints are trochlear, allowing only flexion and extension movement. Hyperextension in the DIP is usual. The capsule of the IP joints is reinforced by the extensor mechanism, the collateral ligaments and the volar plate. Fibres of the proper collateral ligament, which arise dorsal to the axis of the joint thus have an eccentric origin, and become taut as they pass over the flare of the condyle in flexion greater than 60°. Fibres that arise volar to the joint axis, the accessory collateral ligament—volar plate system, are taut in terminal extension (Bowers, 1987a). In the presence of oedema, or collagen rearrangement associated with immobilization, the capsular structure will

Figure 2   Convergence points of the fingers in flexion. Differences are noted in the convergence points of individual finger flexion (a) and simultaneous finger flexion (b). Reproduced from Fess (1989, p. 15).

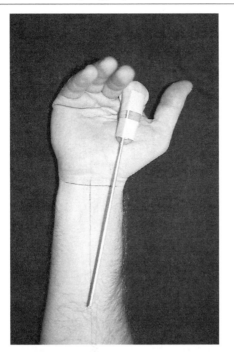

a

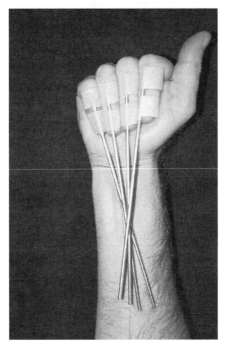

b

tighten further, limiting full extension and full flexion.

The oblique retinacular ligament (ORL), which arises from the volar aspect of the distal third of proximal phalanx, crosses the lateral side of the PIP joint to insert on the distal half of the middle phalanx with fibres intermingling with the distal extensor tendon (Figure 3) (Tubiana *et al.*, 1996). These fibres influence motion of the IP joints. Greater resistance to DIP flexion with the PIP in extension as compared to flexion, is suggestive of abnormal tightness of the ORL. The possibility of contracture in this structure requires consideration in protocols to mobilize the IP joints of the fingers.

Immobilization of joints is commonly used to allow healing of bone and surrounding soft tissue structures. Immobilization positions need to consider the impact of the pathology on the arrangement of capsular, ligamentous and musculotendinous structures.

It is beyond the scope of this anatomical review to describe the complex interconnections between the extrinsic wrist and finger muscles, and the intrinsic finger muscles during motion of the digits. Digital motion is influenced by wrist position with interdependence of muscle action across the three finger joints. For this reason, prior to designing a splint to immobilize, mobilize, or restrict any finger joint motion, careful anatomical analysis is required to determine the implications to both proximal and distal joints, and to adjacent digits. The interconnections between the tendons of the extrinsic muscles, extensor digitorum communis (EDC) and flexor digitorum profundus (FDP), influence the manner in which splints are fabricated to address injuries to these tendons. Interconnections between the EDC tendons, through the junctura on the dor-

Figure 3   A diagrammatic view of the profile of a finger showing insertions of the intrinsic and extrinsic muscles and the retinacular ligaments. 1, Central or middle extensor tendon; 2, lateral extensor tendon; 3, central band of the long extensor; 4, lateral band of the long extensor; 5, interosseous tendon; 6, lumbrical tendon; 7, deep transverse intermetacarpal ligament (or interglenoid); 8, central band of the interosseous; 9, terminal extensor tendon; 10, oblique retinacular ligament; 11, transverse retinacular ligament; 12, triangular ligament; 13, insertion of the extensor digitorum into the second phalanx; 14, transverse fibres of the interosseous hoods; 15, oblique fibres of the interosseous hoods; 16, sagittal bands; 17, fibrous sheath of the flexor tendons; 18, insertion of the interosseous on the base of P_1. 19, tendon of the extensor digitorum; 20, flexor digitorum superficialis; 21, flexor digitorum profundus. Reproduced from Tubiana (1981, p. 53).

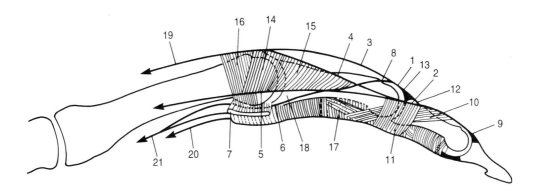

sum of the hand, allow transmission of tension between tendons of adjacent fingers. FDP is one muscle with four tendon units, perhaps with some independence in the index finger. Therefore, protection of one FDP or EDC tendon following tendon repair impacts on motion of the tendons of adjacent digits.

Complex interconnections between the intrinsic and extrinsic musculature through the extensor digital expansion are designed to extend the IP joints. The length relationships are very precise, therefore, swelling, altered bone length and/or adhesions to surrounding tissue, can markedly affect digital function. Differentiating between deficits in extensibility of the intrinsic versus extrinsic musculature is vital to ensure splints target the relevant tissues.

Deformities seen in fingers following paralysis of muscles arising from damage at the spinal cord, brachial plexus or peripheral nerve, or from joint instability or tendon disruption are determined by length, tension and function in residual muscles. Preventing contracture in positions of deformity, and augmenting residual muscle action to gain functional use in areas of paralysis can be achieved by appropriately designed and fabricated splints.

In their path from the forearm to their insertions distally, the tendons are constrained by retinacular ligaments on the volar and dorsal surfaces of the wrist (Figures 4 and 5). A series of pulleys distal to the MCP joints also maintain the finger and thumb flexors close to the phalanges. Retinacular and pulleys are often sites of inflammation. Immobilization or restriction of tendon motion by splints can be used to facilitate healing.

Skin on the palmar surface of the fingers and hand has two primary functions. The first is that of a sensory organ, owing to the enormous number of sensory receptors present. The second function is

Figure 4　The dorsal aspect of the metacarpal and carpometacarpal region of the hand. 1, The interosseous hood; 2, bony insertion of the first dorsal interosseous; 3, extensor indicis; 4, extensor digiti minimi; 5, junctura tendinae; 6, extensor carpi ulnaris; 7, radial artery; 8, extensor carpi radialis longus; 9, extensor carpi radialis brevis; 10, extensor digitorum; 11, extensor retinaculum (dorsal annular ligament of the wrist). Reproduced from De La Caffinière (1981, p. 272).

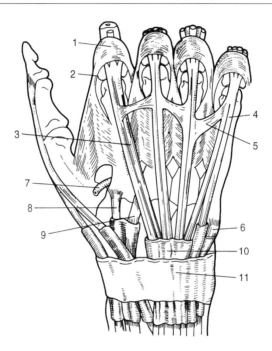

to resist and disperse the very large mechanical forces applied during performance of functional tasks. Volar skin ridges, the adherence of skin to underlying fascia, and the location of fat pads between the digital flexion creases, all contribute to increasing friction and pressure dispersion. Splint design should, therefore, maximize the area on the palmar surface of the fingers and hand available for both sensory and mechanical functions.

Dorsal skin is very mobile with loose connections to underlying tissues. This extensibility is essential to allow movement as the fingers go from extension to flexion. However, thin epidermis and minimal connective tissue elements in the dermis increase the risk of injury should pressure be applied. Nails add support to the pulp and precision to grip. Dynamic splints commonly apply hooks and Velcro® to the nail as a means of securing a force applied to the finger. Application of force to the proximal end is essential to prevent disruption of the nail bed, or modification of nail contour, secondary to sustained pressure.

Clinical experience would suggest that deficits in passive motion in flexion of the MCP, extension of the PIP and flexion of the DIP joints present the greatest therapy challenges in restoring function in the finger ray. These problems can be traced back to the effect of muscle action combined with swelling and contracture of capsular and ligamentous structures.

Figure 5 The relationship of structures on the palmar surface of the hand, particularly flexor tendons, the pulleys, sheaths and the nerves. I, Median nerve; 2, ulnar nerve; the radial (3) and ulnar (4) synovial sheaths of the flexors extend proximally to the wrist. In the fibrous sheaths, note the important mechanical pulleys A_1 and A_2. Reproduced from Tubiana *et al.* (1996, p. 41).

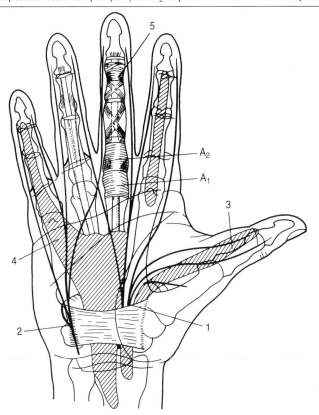

Splints Designed to Immobilize the Fingers

Immobilization of the fingers can be undertaken for a specific joint or several joints within the one digit. The impact of immobilization on proximal and distal joints, and on other digits within the hand must be considered when designing splints and adjunctive therapy programmes.

Splints to Immobilize the Metacarpals

Specific immobilization of the shafts of the metacarpals is undertaken for stable fractures. A hand-based splint may be used in combination with buddy taping to prevent rotation of the fracture and fingers (Figure 6). The location of the opening, whether radial or ulnar, is determined by which finger is injured. Volar and dorsal components apply pressure to minimize any tendency for bone fragments to bow. The volar aspect of the fractured digit is generally longer in order to

Figure 6 Metacarpal immobilization splint. The volar aspect of this splint is extended the length of the fourth metacarpal to ensure greater immobilization of the fractured metacarpal whilst also allowing full motion at other digits. The 'buddy' tape prevents deviation of the proximal phalanx.

Figure 7 Pattern and moulding techniques using plastic-based thermoplastic materials. The size of the piece of splinting material approximates the region of the hand to be splinted. The properties of this plastic-based material are utilized to stretch and mould it to the requirements of this splint.

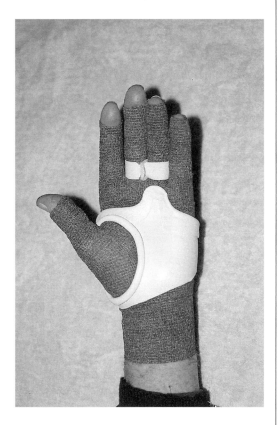

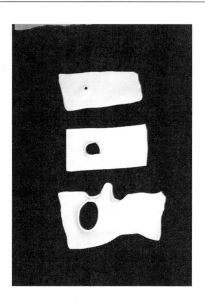

provide better stability acknowledging that flexion has been compromised. Modification of the splint is necessary to maintain the contour of the splint as the swelling resolves.

PATTERN AND FABRICATION PROCEDURE

Precise patterns are not necessary as materials with stretch are used (e.g. Polyform®, Sansplint XR®) (Figure 7). An estimation of the size of material required is based on the lengths of the metacarpals and the circumference of the hand. Immobilization of the index and middle fingers requires a hole to be punched in the centre of the material for the thumb with the opening on the ulnar aspect. For the ring and little fingers, the opening is located on the radial aspect with the hole punched one third from the edge to accommodate the thumb.

The material is heated, the thumb hole created and then the materials moulded to contour the digit involved. When cold, the excess material is marked and then cut. Rolled edges provide strength to the design as well as minimizing shear stress.

Buddy tapes are used to minimize the rotation and some degrees of deviation of the finger. Various designs are described in greater detail in the section on splints that restrict finger motion.

SPLINTS TO IMMOBILIZE MCP, PIP AND DIP JOINTS

Splints that are designed to immobilize an individual finger from either the volar or dorsal surface

Figure 8   MCP, PIP and DIP immobilization splint. The design is circumferential around the hand with a dorsal extension to immobilize the digit. Following surgery to release a Dupuytren's contracture, the finger is immobilized in extension at all joints. Dorsal and volar views are illustrated.

a

b

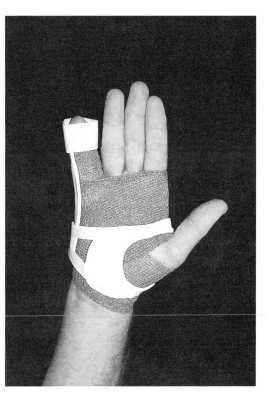

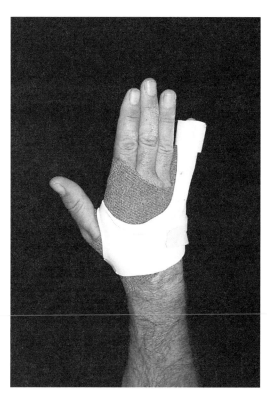

are very similar in design (Figure 8). Materials with stretch are used, therefore, precise patterns are not required. The width is the circumference of the hand. The length is determined by the length of the metacarpals with an extension to include the length of the involved finger ray (Figure 9). The piece of material used is always slightly larger than required to allow for reinforcement. A hole is punched to create access for the thumb. The strength in the finger component is achieved by use of contour. Rolled edges reinforce the narrow component over the MCP joint.

The position of immobilization of the MCP and

PIP joints can vary from full extension, as post-Dupuytren's release, to varying degrees of flexion at the MCP and IP joints, depending on the pathology of the involved tissues. Dorsal application is recommended in the presence of palmar wounds to allow better air circulation around the wound and to allow active and passive flexion exercises without need for removal of the splint.

Splints to Immobilize the PIP Joint

One of the few occasions the PIP joint is immobilized is following injury and repair to the central

Figure 9 Pattern for finger immobilization splints. A precise pattern is not required when splints are manufactured from plastic-based materials. Variations for volar and dorsal designs are illustrated.

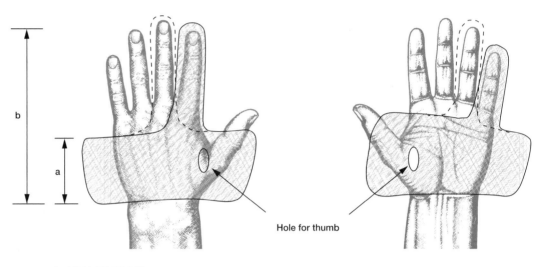

a = length of metacarpals
b = length of involved finger ray

Hole for thumb

slip of the extensor tendon mechanism at the level of the PIP joint. The resultant flexed position of the PIP joint is commonly described as a Boutonniere deformity. Any contracture must be resolved by other forms of splinting prior to immobilization of the joint. Cylindrical splints for the PIP joint are not successful in immobilizing the joint for two reasons. Firstly, the length of the proximal phalanx around which splinting material can be placed is limited, owing to webbing of the skin between digits. Proximal length is, therefore, limited resulting in poor mechanical advantage. Secondly, the soft tissues on the volar surface can be compressed on attempted flexion. Therefore, to achieve sufficient stabilization of the splint on the proximal phalanx, a volar component must be added to extend the splint proximally (Figure 10).

Figure 10 PIP immobilization splint.

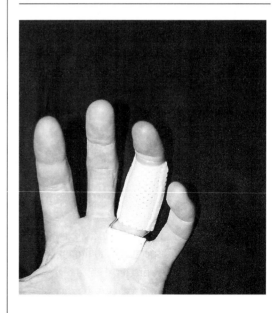

Figure 11   PIP immobilization splint pattern. This splint has good mechanical advantage.

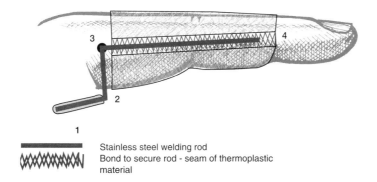

Stainless steel welding rod
Bond to secure rod - seam of thermoplastic material

Fabrication procedure

A cylindrical splint is made with the joint maintained in 0° extension (see Figure 11).

1. A piece of 1.6 mm thickness micro-perforated material is used. The length is determined by the distance between the webspace and the DIP joint. The seam is placed on the lateral aspect of the finger so that it is secured when the base is bonded on. This seam is cut hot.

2. A piece of 1.6 mm stainless steel welding rod (15 cm in length) is used. A U shape in the centre is formed by bending it around a small round object adjusting the width to that of the finger. It is then placed over the proximal end of the phalanx and bent to accommodate the differing lengths identified in Figure 11:

   1–2   Distal palmar crease to proximal digital crease. Note the lengths on the ulnar and radial sides will differ according to finger webbing.

   2–3   Palmar surface to midway between dorsal and palmar aspects of the finger.

   3–4   Length to just proximal to the DIP joint.

A small piece of thermoplastic material is then moulded over the proximal end. The two components are assembled using a thin bond along the length of the welding rod. The therapist should ensure that full motion of the DIP joint is possible. Flexion of the MCP joint is restricted to approximately 60°. The patient is taught to put on and remove the splint whilst the finger is resting on a flat surface so no flexion of the joint occurs.

Splints to Immobilize the DIP Joint

The immobilization of the DIP joint is required following a dorsal fracture of the phalanx distal to the insertion of EDC into the phalanx or rupture of the EDC tendon close to its insertion. This is commonly described as a Mallet deformity. The critical position for a splint used to immobilize the DIP to allow healing of this injury is hyperextension. No pressure should be applied by the splint to the skin on the dorsum of the distal phalanx proximal to the nail (Rayan and Mullins, 1987). Figure 12 illustrates two splints designed to immobilize the distal phalanx. The cylindrical splint provides good positioning; however, it must be altered as the size of the finger changes. Less alteration is required to the second design as the strap and opening along the side of the finger allow the splint to be tightened as the swelling goes down.

Figure 12 DIP immobilization splints. A cylindrical design provides excellent immobilization when the size of the finger does not fluctuate. A design with a lateral opening maintains the finger in the required position whilst allowing adjustment as oedema resolves.

Figure 13 Gentle traction on Theraband® provides hyperextension positioning of the distal phalanx with excellent contour to the volar surface of the splint.

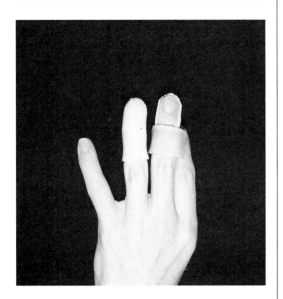

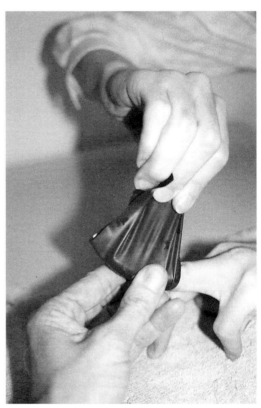

Fabrication procedure

1. A piece of 1.6 mm thermoplastic material the length of the finger distal to the PIP joint and approximately the circumference of the finger is required.

2. Heat the material and place it around the finger. For a circumferential design, place the bond along the dorsal surface. This bond is cut flush with the skin.

3. Position the finger in an extended position by a sling of Theraband® (Figure 13), while applying pressure to position the material around the middle phalanx. Pressure is not applied over the dorsum of the distal phalanx.

4. Remove the splint from the finger while it is sustained against a firm surface in an extended position. Secure the seam with an additional thin strip of splinting material.

5. Ensure that PIP joint flexion is not restricted. Cut off the excess material and very slightly flare the volar surface at the proximal end.

For the open design, the bond is placed along the lateral surface of the digit. On removing it from the finger, split the bond and cut out the dorsal section distal to the DIP joint crease exposing the finger nail. Slightly flare the area along the opening. Small straps are then bonded directly to the splinting material to secure the splint.

Although this splint may look simple, it requires great care to achieve the hyperextended position whilst ensuring the splint is snug but not tight on the finger. Splints must be modified to accommodate changes in swelling in order to maintain the extended position. They are generally worn 24 hours per day for a 6-week period. The critical issue is to educate the client to ensure good skin hygiene, and to maintain the DIP joint in hyper-extension at all times, particularly when putting on and taking off the splint.

Splints Designed to Mobilize the Finger Joints

Mobilization splints fabricated for the fingers address deficits in passive range of motion (ROM). Deficits in extension limit opening of the hand for grasp, while deficits in flexion limit manipulation of objects and power of grasp. Where there are deficits in both extension and flexion within the one digit, priorities must be set to regain that ROM of greatest functional significance to the patient. The expected functional outcome will determine time spent in mobilizing splints. For example, in the stiff hand, gaining flexion to approximately 70° at the PIP joints has precedence over gaining the last 30° of extension. Acknowledging that the ideal is to treat both deficits but being realistic that there are a limited number of hours available for splinting, a 2:1 ratio of flexion:extension splinting may be adopted. The passive ROM (and torque ROM, if available) at the MCP, PIP and DIP joints will determine the type of splinting intervention.

Serial Static Splinting

The choice of material for serial static splinting is determined by the number of digits involved. Plaster is generally used to address IP joint problems owing to its ease of application and low cost, while thermoplastic materials are used to splint the whole hand serially as they are easier to use and remould, and can achieve more precise positioning.

SERIAL STATIC HAND SPLINTS

Various designs are used to address all fingers in the presence of extension deficits, for example, flexor tendon unit tightness. Fabrication requires careful attention to both the wrist and finger positions. Whilst the volar resting splint (see page 89 for pattern details) is commonly used, a splint that has a dorsal forearm component and volar finger component not only increases ease of fabrication, but can distribute force more effectively through splint components as opposed to straps (Figure 14). For the novice therapist, it is often easier to complete fabrication of the wrist and forearm components prior to moulding the finger component to apply gentle tension to the fingers to gain greater extension.

Procedure to take a pattern

1. The length of the splint from wrist to proximal end is two-thirds of the length of the forearm. This roughly equates to the length of the hand. Measure the length using a tape and mark it with a small dot.

2. Position the wrist at an angle close to neutral and allow the fingers and thumb to remain flexed. Lay the pattern material over the dorsum of the hand and mark the following points illustrated in Figure 15a.

   1–2 Medial and lateral aspects of the hand just proximal to the heads of the finger meta-carpals.

Figure 14   Dorsal Volar Hand Splint. This design is used to address extrinsic flexor tendon tightness or extension deficits in the joints of multiple fingers. An extension force is applied to the palmar surface of the fingers. (top) Finger position is maintained by finger loops, threaded through a flat ring of thermoplastic material (or 'D' ring) on the volar surface. (bottom) Loops are lengthened to get into the splint then secured flush with each digit.

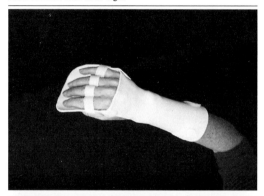

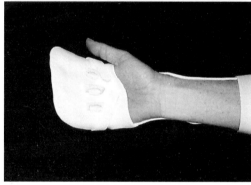

3–4 Medial and lateral aspects of the hand at the thumb web level.

5–6 Medial and lateral aspects of the wrist at mid-carpal level.

7–8 Medial and lateral aspects of the forearm at the length previously determined.

9   The index middle finger web.

Allowance is added to support the side of the little finger (2a). The width of the splint should be half the circumference at the forearm and wrist. This can be determined by wrapping the pattern material around and marking the desired width at the forearm and wrist. These width points are indicated on the diagram as 6a, 8a, etc.

The volar finger component extends from the heads of metacarpals to the tips of the fingers. Place the pattern material under the client's fingers with the wrist in some flexion so that the fingers can be extended. Mark the medial and lateral aspects of the hand just proximal to the heads of the finger metacarpals as illustrated in Figure 15c. The finger component should be slightly longer than the fingers.

To shape the pattern, see Figure 15b:

1. Join points 1 and 2 (MCP line).
2. Join points 3–4 (thumb line).
3. Join points 5–6 (wrist line).
4. Draw a vertical line from point 9 to intersect the wrist line.
5. Starting at point 2a, draw a line around the forearm through points 4a, 6a and 8a, curve sharply around to 7a then up to 5. The curve through 7a should be shallow to ensure this aspect of the splint does not impede elbow flexion.
6. The line between 5 and 3 touches the vertical line 9 allowing clearance for thumb tendons.
7. Points 1 and 3 are joined.
8. Cut the two pattern pieces out. When fitted to the hand, the proximal edge of the palmar component is aligned to the thumb line of the dorsal component. Check for fit on the patient prior to transferring it to the thermoplastic material. Pad out the ulna head using a small piece of exercise putty.

Fabrication procedure Prior to fabricating this splint, it is important to determine the angle at which the wrist and the MCP joints are to be immobilized.

1. The arm should be positioned with the elbow supported, and the wrist in the predeter-

Figure 15   Dorsal volar hand splint pattern.

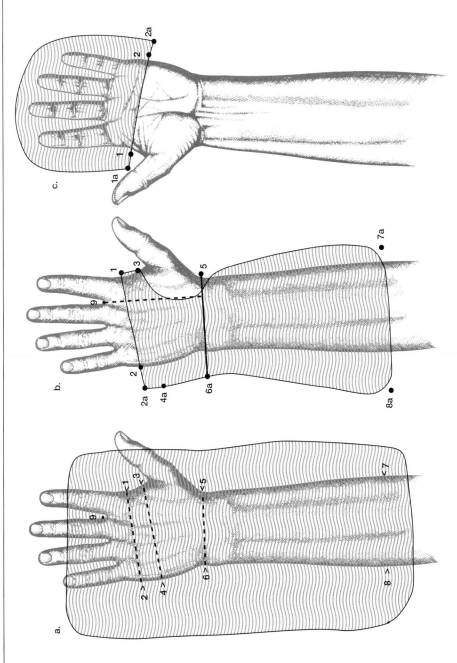

mined position. Do not be concerned with the finger position when moulding the forearm component.

2. Remove the forearm component from the heating source and apply to the patient's hand and secure it in place. Mould intimately around the wrist, the arches of the hand, and gently flare the proximal and distal ends and around the thumb.

3. When the forearm component is completely cold, the palmar component is attached. The wrist is flexed so that full extension can be achieved with the fingers. The wrist component remains in place on the dorsum of the hand. The palmar component is positioned under the fingers with the sides turned up to bond on to the dorsal component on the sides of the index and little finger metacarpal heads.

4. Once the bonds are secure, the fingers are positioned in the degrees of MCP flexion previously determined. IP joints are held in extension.

5. A strap is attached at the proximal end of the forearm at the wrist and, if necessary, over the proximal phalanx of the fingers to prevent flexion.

To increase the extension of the fingers, only the palmar component need be modified until the neutral position of the IP joints of the fingers is achieved. Then the MCP joint position is gradually extended in combination with the wrist.

Securing each finger by a loop threaded through the palmar component will ensure the position is maintained. A small slit is made between the fingers. The strap is threaded through the hole, through a securing loop on the volar surface and then back through the same slit. Thus, one strap secures all fingers. The sides of the splint should not be higher than the fingers so that the strap sits flush with the dorsum of the index and little fingers.

SERIAL STATIC FINGER CASTS

Serial casting is recommended for resolution of IP joint contractures where there is significant pain or chronic inflammation, when contractures are long standing, or to maximize total end range time (TERT) and compliance. Plaster casting involves gentle positioning of the contracted tissue near the end of its elastic limit for 24 hours per day, that is, maximal TERT. Bell (1987) states that 'no force greater than that which would be used to extend the tissue is applied' (p. 454). Casts are generally applied for periods of 3–5 days. On removal of the cast, active and passive movements through the available range of motion are undertaken to prevent complications of prolonged immobilization. A new cast is then applied in the new lengthened position. Four or five casts are applied, with casting ceasing when the desired ROM is reached or when other forms of mobilizing splinting can be used.

Fabrication procedure

1. Very small amounts of cotton wool can be used to minimize shear between skin and plaster over the dorsum of the PIP joint. Alternatively, a single layer of wax (as used in the wax bath) can be painted strategically over the PIP joint. As the plaster is setting, the heat melts the wax that impregnates the plaster bandage creating a smooth area.

2. Small plaster bandage strips, 2 cm in width and between 20–25 cm in length, are rolled into small bandages. Prepare a minimum of two per finger.

3. Neat smooth edges are achieved on the proximal and distal ends of the cast by turning 5 mm over to form a small hem on the plaster bandage.

Figure 16 Spiral wrapping of narrow plaster bandage around the finger provides a neat but strong cast.

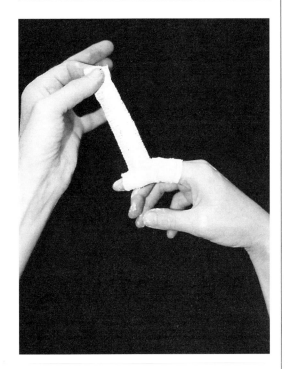

4. The finger is positioned and the plaster dipped into luke warm water and then applied to the finger without tension. A complete wrap is made around the proximal end prior to overlapping by half as it is wrapped distally around the digit. Inclusion of the DIP joint will be determined by pathology. Two applications of plaster bandage are all that is necessary (Figure 16).

5. To position the finger, the therapist holds the MCP and the distal phalanx over the nail and gently extends the finger until the plaster becomes warm and sets firmly. Slight traction may also be applied by the patient resting their finger in a cradle of Theraband® (Figure 13).

6. Smooth all the edges and surfaces of the cast.

7. The plaster can be removed by soaking it in water. Should pain and discomfort arise, the patient should be instructed to soak off the plaster.

If active motion is not able to sustain gains in range of motion, other forms of static splinting should be considered after casting. Application during non-functional times of the day is recommended.

Dynamic Splints

In designing splints to address passive ROM deficits in the finger joints, consideration must be given to the length of the base. Splints that include the wrist provide secure anchorage, a larger area for pressure dispersion, and the potential for the use of multiple outriggers and longer traction. However, these advantages must be weighed against immobilization of proximal joints, and compliance issues that are associated with larger splints. Splints traversing the wrist are used for multiple digit problems, where ROM deficits pertain to extrinsic musculotendinous adhesions, and when deficits in both flexion and extension are to be addressed within the one splint. Hand-based designs are generally used for single digit or single joint problems.

Dynamic splints require regular review so that the direction of force remains at the correct angle and tension created by the elastic bands is not diminished by material fatigue. After initial fabrication, the patient should be seen within 2–3 days to determine the response of the tissues to the force applied, and then on a regular basis thereafter.

SPLINT DESIGNS TO MOBILIZE THE MCP JOINT

Owing to its capsular and ligamentous arrangement, the MCP joint will generally contract in extension. A deficit in flexion of the MCP joint

Figure 17 Dynamic MCP extension splint. A dorsal wrist immobilization splint with an extended palmar bar forms the basis of this splint.

Figure 18 Dynamic MCP Flexion Splint. The functional deficit for this adolescent girl with Scleroderma is the lack of MCP joint flexion not the PIP joint flexion contractures. A dynamic flexion splint applied 10 hours per day for 8 months required excellent compliance.

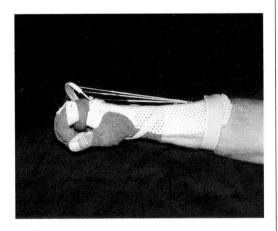

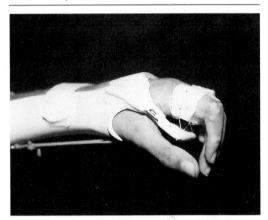

has a profound impact on the ability to achieve a gross grasp as well as opposition for pinch. Contracture of this joint is often associated with paralysis of intrinsic musculature, inappropriate immobilization subsequent to wrist casting or the presence of significant pain when the hand is immobilized. Resolution of contracture tends to be aided by functional use of the hand after approximately 45° flexion. Flexion contracture of the MCP joints is seen, but generally associated with conditions that impact upon other joints and structures in the hand. The flexion and ulnar deviation deformity of the MCP joints, seen in rheumatoid arthritis, is most commonly splinted following joint reconstructive surgery (Figure 17).

Wrist immobilization splints (described in Chapter 5) form the base of finger mobilizing splints that require a long base to secure an outrigger and traction. The circumferential design is most commonly used as a base for splints addressing deficits in MCP flexion (Figures 2 and 3 in Chapter 9), while the dorsal design with an extended palmar component (Figures 12 and 13 in Chapter 5) is used for deficits in MCP extension. To fabricate the

splint, the base component is made in the usual manner. The straps are attached and secured prior to determining the position and angle of the outrigger. In the presence of flexion deficits in the index MCP joint, the thumb is positioned in a more extended position to allow room for the outrigger. The outrigger must accommodate the unique angle of pull for each digit. The procedure to determine the shape and the position of the outrigger is described in Chapter 3, page 60. The pull should always be at 90° to the longitudinal axis of the proximal phalanx.

Hand-based splints (Figure 20) use a circumferential design, not involving the thumb. The pattern for the base is similar to that illustrated in Figure 9 with dimensions varying according to the digital length required. Consideration is given to the location of the outrigger in determining the position of the opening and the straps.

SPLINT DESIGNS TO MOBILIZE THE PIP JOINT

The design of dynamic splints to mobilize the PIP joint is determined firstly by the number of digits

Figure 19   Sustained low load dynamic splinting over an 8 month period gained sufficient MCP range for the finger tips to touch the palm for effective grip.

Figure 20   Hand-based dynamic MCP flexion splint. When one or two digits have a deficit in MCP flexion, a hand-based splint will allow application of traction to achieve the desired range.

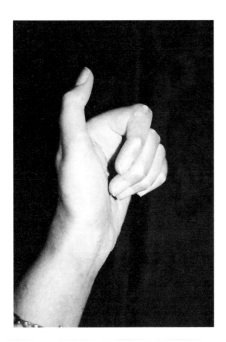

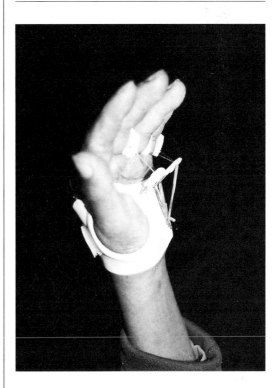

involved. Splints that use springs can address only one joint, whilst hand- and forearm-based splints with traction components can address multiple digits and deficits in multiple directions.

Capner splint is the common name for the dynamic PIP extension splint where the force is generated by spring wire (Capner, 1967) (Figure 21). Custom-made splints ensure better fit and comfort. However, the prefabricated designs (see Figure 30) available from splinting suppliers are recommended over choosing not to splint owing to an inability to overcome the challenges of splint fabrication. This splint is used to address deficits in extension of the PIP joint less than 45°. Thin non-perforated material is used for the moulded components of this splint. Thermoplastic components have advantages over soft tape.

The moulded thermoplastic ensures intimate contact with changing dimensions of the finger, particularly in the vicinity of the PIP joint, which is often enlarged. It also ensures that the longitudinal alignment of the springs is maintained over the narrower distal phalanx, thereby minimizing rotation and preventing the patient adjusting the force applied.

However, the moulded thermoplastic may be placed on the dorsum of the finger and a Velcro® loop used to secure the finger to the splint. This design may be used in the presence of greater degrees of PIP contracture or when dimensions or sensitivity of the finger may make application of the splint difficult.

Figure 21   Dynamic PIP extension (Capner) splints. Pressure to extend the PIP is applied by a Velcro® strap in the ring finger, and a thermoplastic sling in the middle finger. When multiple splints are applied the size of the palmar component is adjusted. Dorsal and volar views.

a

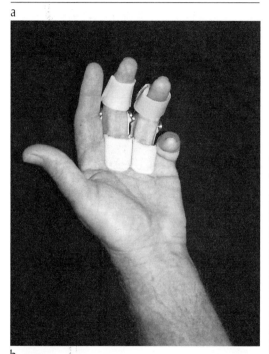

b

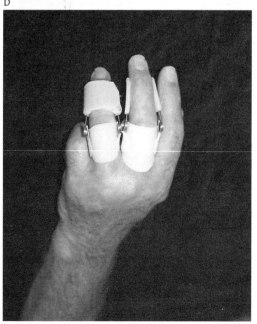

Fabrication procedure Springs can be made or purchased ready made from splinting material suppliers. Start with a piece of spring wire (gauge 13), length 15 cm. Two tight complete coils of equal diameter are located one-third from the end. A simple jig (available from splinting suppliers) is used to coil springs, one in a clockwise and the other an anticlockwise direction. The spring arms should be horizontal for a 0° end range of force and aligned longitudinally. The spring is positioned at the axis of the PIP joint with the spring arm distal and then bent according to the lengths illustrated in Figure 22.

1–2   Length from PIP joint to the web of the digit.

2–3   Height midway between the dorsal and palmar aspects of the finger and the palmar surface.

3–4   Length from the finger web to the proximal palmar crease. Note the lengths on the ulnar and radial sides will differ according to finger webbing.

1–5   Length from PIP joint to just proximal to the DIP joint. This length may be longer if the splint traverses this joint. It is important to remember that the torque at the PIP joint will differ depending on where

Figure 22   Pattern for a PIP dynamic extension splint. Spring wire is curled into a spring and then bent to accommodate finger dimensions.

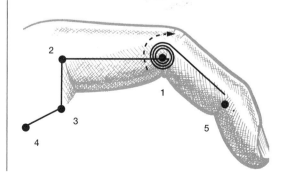

the force is applied on the middle phalanx or distal phalanx.

Fabrication procedure

1. A very small component of both ends of the spring is bent across the palm at the proximal end, and volarly at the distal end, to ensure the sharp end faces away from the patient's skin.

2. The dorsal hood is made from a piece of 1.6 mm material moulded over the dorsal aspect of the proximal phalanx.

3. The springs are aligned to the PIP joint and the position marked on the dorsal hood. The edges of the material is reheated and folded securing the spring.

4. The small piece of material is moulded over the wires to form the palmar component and to maintain the finger width.

5. The splint is then fitted to the finger and the final loop moulded to the volar surface of the middle phalanx, or middle and distal phalanges. Align the distal arm of the springs and mark the location on the splinting material. Reheat the edges and fold the splinting material over the wire. Alternatively, the splinting material is placed over the dorsum of the finger to secure the spring arms. A Velcro® loop is then attached to this piece of splinting material, allowing the patient to adjust the force applied.

An alternative procedure to fabricate this splint from one piece of spring wire with soft attachments to the wire made of filament tape, moleskin and Velcro® is described in Colditz (1995).

In order to apply an effective force to mobilize the PIP joint in a hand-based splint, it is essential that the proximal phalanx is immobilized with a reactive force to prevent the proximal phalanx moving within the confines of the splint. In the presence of extension deficits, this is best achieved by volar

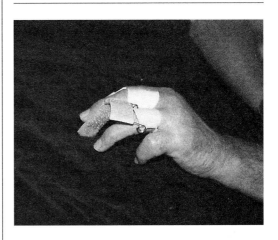

Figure 23 PIP dynamic extension splint with a volar strap. The application of a strap, as opposed to a moulded thermoplastic component, allows easier access and more adjustment to the force applied by the spring.

and dorsal components effectively sandwiching the proximal phalanx as illustrated in Figure 24. For a flexion deficit in a single digit a volar component with a dorsal strap is sufficient.

The patterns used for these splints are the same as those used to immobilize the finger (Figure 9). Ensure that the length of the pattern is adjusted for the finger component to accommodate increased dorsal length as the MCP is flexed. The location of the outrigger is considered in positioning the opening and the straps. The procedure to determine the shape and the position of the outrigger is described in Chapter 3, page 60.

SPLINT DESIGNS TO MOBILIZE THE DIP JOINT

Deficits in motion of the DIP joint are not uncommon with lack of flexion having the greatest impact on function. Where flexion is less than 45°, a finger-based splint is recommended. Effective immobilization of the PIP joint means all the torque is directed to the DIP joint. The base to this splint is that used to immobilize the PIP joint

Figure 24 Dynamic PIP extension splint. Dynamic traction is applied via a series of low-profile outriggers to three fingers with differing deficits in ROM (top). The volar view illustrates blocking of the proximal phalanges to control with reactive forces (bottom).

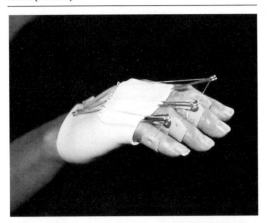

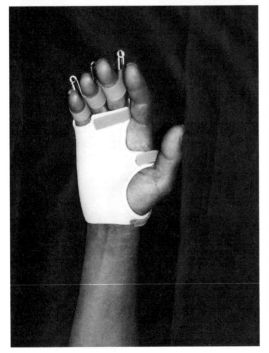

Figure 25 Dynamic PIP flexion splint. Similar deficits in motion in flexion of the PIP joints are addressed by traction directed through a single outrigger.

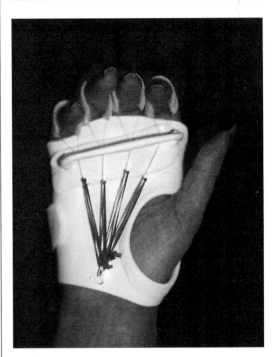

described in Figures 10 and 11. A small outrigger made from a safety pin is attached to direct the correct line of pull to a hook secured over the palmar component (Figure 26).

Deficits in DIP flexion are often a consequence of injury to the PIP joint. Addressing end range flexion at both joints can be achieved by a small splint that consists of two parts (Figure 27). A thimble, of very thin thermoplastic material, is made over the distal phalanx with a small dress hook secured over the tip. The second component is moulded over the dorsal surface of the proximal phalanx with the PIP joint in maximum flexion. A small elastic band is attached to the hook and taken over the dorsum of the proximal phalanx. A small block made of splinting material prevents this band changing alignment. Tolerance to wearing DIP flexion splints is generally not greater than 1 hour. Therefore, repeated applications are recommended to maximize end range time.

Figure 26   Dynamic DIP flexion splint. Traction applied to the DIP joint requires good immobilization of the PIP joint. A safety pin forms the outrigger and a dress hook anchorage for the traction.

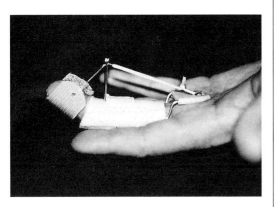

Figure 27   Dynamic DIP / PIP flexion splint. A thimble made of thermoplastic material over the distal phalanx anchors traction applied from the dorsum of the proximal phalanx to flex the PIP and DIP joints simultaneously.

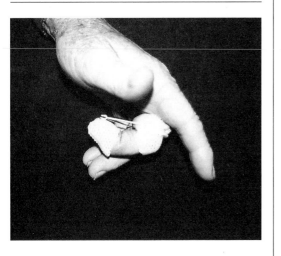

Figure 28   Dynamic finger flexion splint. A single loop anchored to the fingernail applies a flexion force affecting all finger joints. This design is appropriate if there are deficits in motion in all joints.

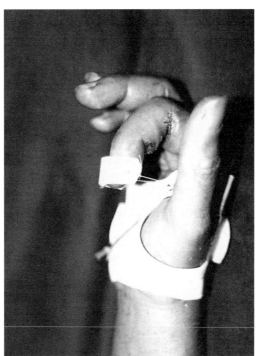

should be directed specifically to each joint. Figure 29 illustrates a splint with a force directed to the MCP via the proximal phalanx, and then a second applied to the fingernail to effect motion at the PIP and DIP. Hand-based splints may be used for a single finger but forearm-based splints are recommended where multiple fingers are to be splinted.

MULTIPLE JOINT DYNAMIC SPLINT DESIGNS

When all joints of the finger have similar deficits in passive joint flexion, a splint designed to effect motion at all three joints can be used (Figure 28). However, if the mobility of successive joints is not similar, the line of pull of the dynamic traction

PREFABRICATED DYNAMIC FINGER SPLINTS

Numerous prefabricated dynamic finger splints are available (Figure 30). Their advantage is that no splint fabrication skills are required, and the cost of time for fabrication and application is minimal. The disadvantage of these splints is that

Figure 29   Dynamic finger flexion splint. Individual finger loops and outriggers are necessary when limitation in joint motion is not equal in successive joints.

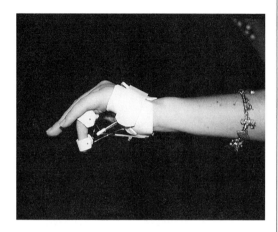

Figure 30   Prefabricated PIP extension splints. LMB finger springs are one brand of prefabricated finger splints (LMB Hand Rehab Products, P.O. Box 1181, San Luis Obispo, CA 93406, USA).

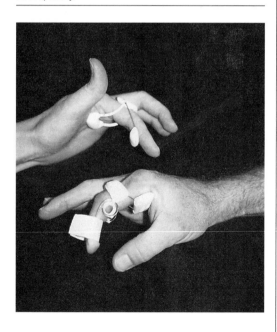

the location of the axis of the splint often does not match the axis of joint, with other components not matching the size of the finger. However, for therapists without the skill or resources to fabricate dynamic finger splints, prefabricated splints can be used to fulfil therapeutic objectives for increasing range of motion.

Splints Designed to Restrict Motion in the Finger Joints

Splints designed to restrict motion in a finger are used to protect healing structures, particularly ligaments and tendons, or to redirect active motion of non-paralysed muscles to effect motion in targeted joints. When restricting finger joints to facilitate healing, the surface of application dictates the motion to be limited. Dorsal application will limit extension, volar application flexion, and medial or lateral application will restrict deviation.

Facilitate Healing

There are many protocols for the post-operative rehabilitation of finger flexor and extensor tendon repairs. The reader is referred to recent reviews by Stewart and van Strien (1995) and Evans (1995) on flexor and extensor tendon repairs respectively, for more detailed information on management protocols. Within each protocol a form of restrictive splint is used with the specific angles of joint position varying.

DORSAL WRIST AND HAND SPLINT (FINGER FLEXOR TENDON REPAIRS)

A dorsal hand splint is used to restrict the range of extension of the fingers, whilst allowing either passive, active, or active and passive digital motion into flexion (Figure 31). The wrist is immobilized between 10° and 40° flexion, the MCP joints between 30° and 60° flexion, with the IP joints

Figure 31   Dorsal wrist and finger extension block splint. The basic component of all protocols for management of finger flexor tendon repairs is a splint, which immobilizes the wrist and blocks MCP joint extension. An extended palmar bar is hinged by straps to allow excellent access to the splint. The addition of straps and dynamic traction components is dependent upon the protocol used.

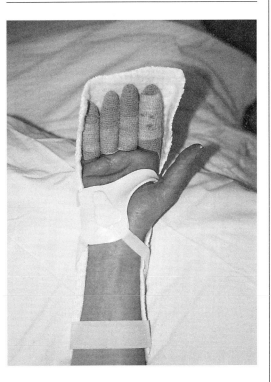

allowed to assume full extension. A moulded palmar component is recommended when fabricating the splint to support the transverse arch and decrease potential for flexion to occur at either the wrist or the MCP joints.

Procedure to take a pattern

1. Position the patient's hand in a safe position. In the presence of flexor tendon repairs, it is advisable to support the wrist in flexion and between neutral and 10° ulnar deviation, with the fingers and thumb completely relaxed. Place the pattern material over the dorsum of the hand.

2. The length of the splint from wrist to proximal end is generally two-thirds the length of the forearm. This roughly equates to the length of the hand. Measure the length using a tape and mark it with a small dot.

Mark the following points as illustrated in Figure 32:

1–2   Medial and lateral aspects of the hand just proximal to the heads of the finger metacarpals.

3–4   Medial and lateral aspects of the wrist at mid-carpal level.

5–6   Medial and lateral aspects of the forearm at the length previously determined.

7   Length of the middle finger.

8   Between the index and middle finger web.

The width of the splint should be half the circumference at the forearm and wrist. This can be determined by wrapping the pattern material around and marking the desired width at the forearm, wrist and MCP joints. These width points are indicated on the diagram as 1a, 2a, 4a, etc.

To shape the pattern

1. Join points 1 and 2 (MCP line) and 3–4 (wrist line).

2. Draw a vertical line from point 8 to intersect the wrist line. This line is used as a guide to allow movement of the thumb.

3. Starting at point 7, draw a line connecting 2a, 4a and 6a, curve sharply around to 5a then up to 3. The curve through 5a should be shallow to ensure this aspect of the splint does not impede elbow flexion. The line between 3 and 1a allows for movement of the thumb in extension.

4. Cut the pattern out. If the splinting material does not have a high degree of stretch and drape, it is necessary to make a small dart on either side of the MCP joints. Cut the material

Figure 32 Pattern for a dorsal wrist and finger splint.

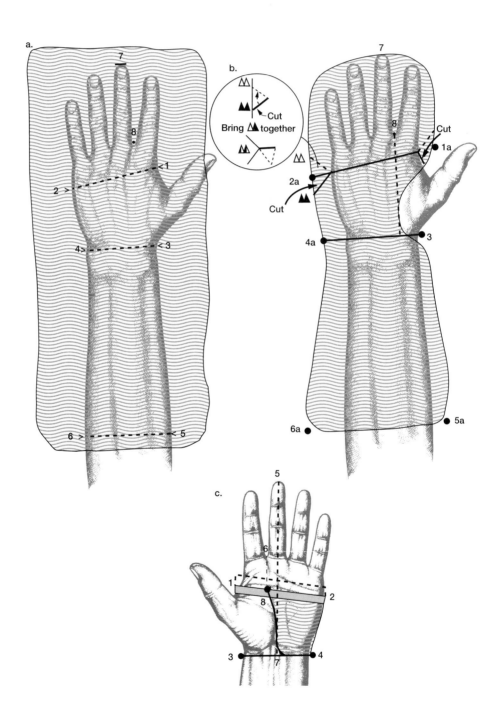

on the medial and lateral aspects of the MCP joints (as illustrated in the circle in Figure 32b) to reposition the dorsal finger component into flexion. Check for fit on the patient, ensuring the forearm is maintained in a pronated position, prior to transferring it to the thermoplastic material. Ensure the extensor action of extensor pollicus longus in not compromised by the splint distal to its exit from the extensor retinaculum.

5. Transfer the pattern to splinting material.

A separate volar component is used to contact the volar surface of the hand for support of the arches and dispersion of pressure. It is possible to incorporate this into the dorsal component and cut it out as one piece of thermoplastic material. Mark the following points with reference to Figure 32c.

1–2 Medial and lateral aspects of the hand just proximal to the heads of the finger metacarpals.

3–4 Wrist at the radiocarpal level.

5 Tip of the middle finger.

6 The index and middle finger web.

To shape the pattern:

1. Join points 1 and 2 (MCP line).

2. Join points 3–4 (wrist line).

3. Draw a vertical line from point 5 to intersect the wrist line – point 7.

4. Draw a vertical line from point 6 to intersect the MCP line – point 8. These lines are used as a guide to determine the location of the thenar crease.

5. Draw a line from 2 to 4, then across the wrist to point 7.

6. The line between 7 and 8 follows the thenar crease.

Fabrication procedure

1. The arm should be positioned with the elbow supported, the forearm in a vertical position in mid-pronation–supination, and the wrist supported in the predetermined position. Allow room for the changing dimensions of the distal ulna by padding out the ulna head prior to fabrication.

2. Remove the thermoplastic material from the heating source. If necessary, make darts to accommodate flexion angle at the MCP joints.

3. Apply the material to the patient's hand and secure it to the forearm with a bandage if necessary. Mould intimately around the wrist, the dorsum of the hand and the MCP joints, and gently flare around the thumb and the distal end. It is important to achieve the desired angle of flexion of the MCP joints by intimately moulding the splinting material across the metacarpals and proximal phalanges. Care must be taken to mould the splint over the dorsum of the fingers without applying any stress to the fingers.

4. Mould the separate hand component with the dorsal splint in place. Cut, then heat the splinting material. Gently roll the distal palmar end and around the thenar crease to provide a smooth surface. Mould to the hand ensuring that movement of the finger MCP joints and thumb is not compromised. The palmar component should contour well to the arches of the hand.

5. Straps are used to secure the palmar component to the dorsal component on the ulnar and radial aspects. Hook Velcro® is attached to the volar component with pile Velcro® attached to the dorsal component. The ulnar strap can be attached permanently to both splint components to act as a hinge for ease of access. An

additional strap is located at the proximal end of the splint.

DORSAL HAND SPLINT (FINGER EXTENSOR TENDON REPAIRS)

Extensor tendons repaired in zones V–VII are generally splinted with a dynamic extension traction that maintains the finger MCP joints in a 0° extended position (Evans, 1995). The splint has a dorsal forearm component that positions the wrist in an extended position, while the palmar component restricts flexion to predetermined angles.

The pattern is the same as that used for the static serial hand splint (Figure 15). During the pattern taking and fabrication procedure, the fingers must be supported in extension at all times.

1. The dorsal forearm component is moulded first with the patient supporting the fingers.
2. The straps are then applied to the forearm component so that they can secure this part of the splint to the forearm while the finger component is made.
3. The palmar component is heated, positioned

Figure 33   Dynamic MCP extension splint with a flexion block. A combined dorsal volar hand splint is the base for a dynamic splint used in the management of finger extensor tendon repairs.

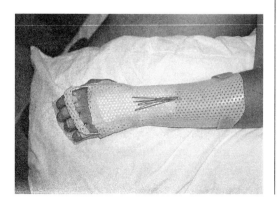

on the hand and bonded on the medial and lateral surfaces of the dorsal component. MCP joint flexion is adjusted to the predetermined angle initially around 30°.
4. The outrigger is bent to accommodate the fingers suspended in a zero position at the MCP joints. The procedure to determine the shape and position of the outrigger is described in Chapter 3, page 60.
5. The length and tension of the elastic traction is determined using the formula described on page 57.

The patient is required to flex to the palmar component actively and let the traction return the fingers to a zero position. Gradually, over the period of 6 weeks, the angle of MCP flexion is increased, with the palmar component cut down to allow for greater PIP and DIP joint flexion.

HAND- AND FINGER-BASED SPLINTS TO RESTRICT FINGER MOTION

Hand-based splints that restrict motion of the finger joints are used for isolated digit injuries that do not involve repaired tendons (Figure 34). Extension block splinting as it is commonly described is used for certain fracture dislocations of the PIP joints, and following repair to the volar plate or digital nerves. The pattern and procedures for fabrication are illustrated in Figure 9 and described on page 120. The amount of restriction in motion at each of the finger joints is determined by the pathology.

Restriction of medial and lateral motion of the MCP and PIP joints, while still allowing flexion and extension, is achieved by coupling the involved finger to its non-involved neighbour by what is commonly described as a 'buddy tape'. The non-injured finger can provide both support and passive motion during functional movements of the

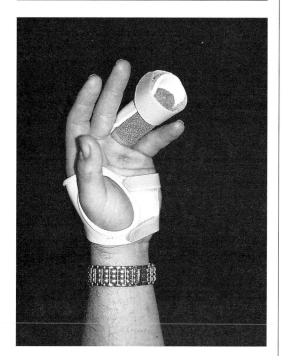

Figure 34 Dorsal extension blocking splints. The pathology will determine the degree of restriction at the MCP, PIP and DIP joints. A position of 70° MCP flexion with IP extension is used for digital nerve repairs, while flexion of both MCP and PIP joints is required following volar plate injuries.

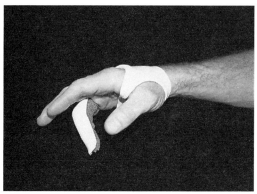

fingers. The length discrepancy of ulnar digits requires the loops for each finger to be offset otherwise flexion of the digits is compromised. Bowers (1987b) cautions that there is a risk of undesirable rotational forces occurring in the

injured finger forced to track in tandem with its neighbour. Where this risk is present, splinting should be specifically directed to the involved joint.

Buddy tapes can be manufactured from Velcro®. The simplest design requires a length of Velcro® equal to the circumference of the involved fingers plus 2.5 cm (Figure 35a). Narrow Velcro® is recommended. A small hole is cut 0.5 cm from one end. With the pile side towards the inside, the end is threaded through the hole and looped around the adjacent finger. Hook Velcro® sewn to the dorsal aspect secures the loop. Alternatively, a small piece of hook Velcro® is sewn to a longer length of pile Velcro®. Both textured surfaces are orientated in the same direction so that the pile can attach to the hook as it is brought around the finger. The little finger generally requires the loops to be offset to accommodate different positions of the phalanges (Figure 35b).

Restricting hyperextension or medial or lateral deviation of the PIP joint can be achieved with a small splint (Figure 36). This design does not impede other functions of the PIP joint. The splint used to resolve both deformities requires a piece of thin splinting material cut according to Figure 37. Orfit® 1.6 mm non-perforated material is recommended for this splint. The tendency for Aquaplast® to shrink slightly when cooling can lead to constriction of the finger if care is not taken during moulding.

Length is determined by the distance from the webspace to the DIP joint, with the width at least half the circumference of the finger. Two large holes are punched.

1. Hand cream is applied to the slightly flexed finger to ensure the material slides on easily.
2. On removing material from the heating source, stretch the holes slightly. Place the finger

Figure 35 'Buddy-tape' splints. (a) 'Buddy-tape' configuration made of a single piece of Velcro® is appropriate when adjacent fingers are the same length. (b) 'Buddy' tape for the little finger generally requires two loops which are then stitched together.

Figure 36 PIP extension blocking splint. Hyperextension deformity secondary to a volar plate injury at the PIP joint is managed by a splint which restricts PIP joint hyperextension without compromise to other joint function.

a

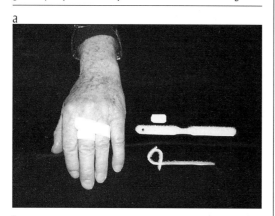

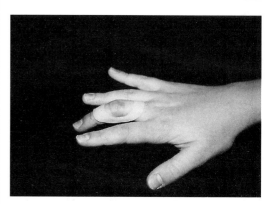

b

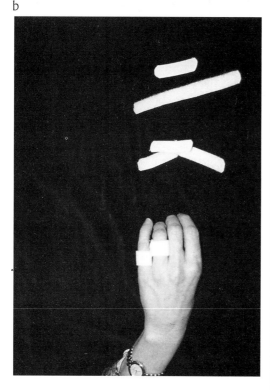

through the holes and move the material down the finger being careful not to overstretch it.

3. The sides are folded volarly and well contoured against the side of the digit.

4. This splint is removed from the finger when the material is *completely cold*. The edges are then trimmed to ensure no material extends beyond the volar surface of the finger.

5. If necessary, the volar bar is rolled to decrease its width across the PIP joint as flexion should not be compromised.

For persons with a permanent deformity, a more acceptable solution is the use of custom-made ring splints. These are manufactured in silver and can be ordered from the Silver Ring Splint Company (P.O. Box 2856, Charlottesville, VA22902–2856, USA) or manufactured to specification by jewellers.

MCP DEVIATION SPLINTS

The deviation of the fingers in an ulnar direction presents a splinting challenge to the very experienced therapist. Correction of the deformity can be achieved in a volar resting splint. However, it is during performance of functional tasks that limitations become evident. Identification of the problem by the patient is critical if a splint to correct the deformity is to be worn. Advantages

Figure 38   Pattern for a PIP extension block splint.

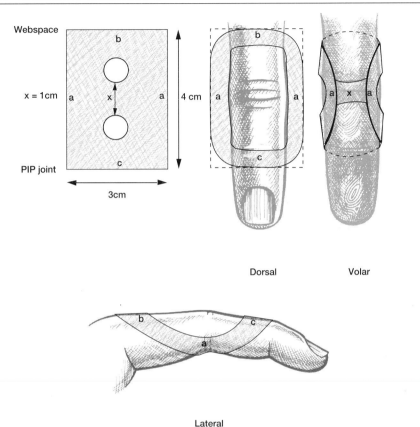

Dorsal   Volar

Lateral

of the splint in positioning the fingers for function have to be weighed against the presence of splinting materials in the hand (Rennie, 1996). Many prefabricated styles are available but tend to be bulky.

Splints to Facilitate Functional Muscle Action

Where damage to the median and/or ulnar nerve has occurred within the vicinity of the wrist, extrinsic muscle action predominates in the fingers, resulting in deformities that are exacerbated by resisted motion of the fingers. Paralysis of the interossei and lumbricals results in flexion of the DIP and PIP joints with extension at the MCP joints, described as an intrinsic minus position. This impacts on grasp owing to the inability to extend the IP joints, limiting the size of objects grasped. To overcome this deformity, restriction of extension of the MCP joints allows the full action of FDP and FDS to effect IP flexion, and EDC to extend the IP joints through its interconnections in the extensor hood (Figure 38). Clinical experience suggests that many splints designed to address this deformity are discarded by patients as the deficits associated with their use are greater than the benefits. When the patient identifies an occupational task where finger function would be

Figure 38 An ulnar nerve palsy splint. Blocking hyperextension at the MCP joint will facilitate functional extension of the IP joints following ulnar nerve paralysis.

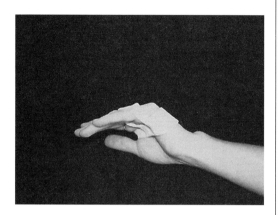

enhanced by a restricting extension, a simple splint is recommended.

The splint requires anchorage to the palm of the hand. An additional piece of material is moulded across the dorsum of the involved fingers to prevent extension of the MCP joints. Ideally, the splint components should be thin; however, if they are too thin, they will move and rotate on the hand creating discomfort.

This splint is manufactured from two pieces of splinting material. To prevent rotation of the splint on the hand, the material that traverses the dorsum is slightly wider than the component across the palm. The width of the material is determined by the size of the hand. The length equals the circumference of the hand.

1. The material is intimately moulded to contours of the hand just proximal to the heads of the metacarpals. The join is placed on the ulnar aspect of the hand and cut hot to ensure a smooth bond.

2. The fingers are then positioned in flexion at the MCP joints. A second piece of material is adhered to the palmar bar on the ulnar aspect of the hand over the seam, taken over the dorsum of the fingers and then adhered back to the palmar bar on the radial aspect. Contour is especially important over the dorsum of the fingers.

3. When only the ring and little fingers are involved, the piece of material through the webspace of the middle and ring fingers should not create pressure or cause friction with movement.

4. All edges are gently flared to avoid pressure.

Splints to Optimize Function

In situations where paralysis impairs the ability to grasp and position objects in the hand, splints may be used. These splints are generally performance specific, in that they secure an object, such as a pen, an eating utensil, or a joystick so that proximal limb function can be used to achieved the functional objective.

Writing is an important functional task and information on fabrication of this splint is used to illustrate how the splinting materials can be used for this objective. Figure 39 illustrates the writing splint and two stages in its fabrication.

A narrow piece of splinting material is required approximately the circumference of the thumb and index and middle fingers. The heated material is wound around the pen at a slight angle, with approximately one-third the length allowed for the thumb. The pen is then positioned on the fingers, and the short component wound around the thumb and joined to the splinting material on the volar aspect of the pen. The longer component is wound around the fingers and joined to the pen. Any additional material is cut off. Sustain the correct position of the pen, ensuring that it

Figure 39 Writing splint. Three stages in the fabrication are illustrated. The thermoplastic material wound around the pen, the completed loop for the thumb, and the splint with loops around the fingers and thumb, ensuring that the pen is orientated to touch the paper.

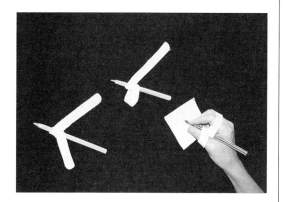

can contact the paper, and mould to the contours of the fingers and thumb.

Conclusion

The function of the hand is dependent on movement and stability of the fingers for fine dexterity in addition to transmission of force in object and tool manipulation. Mobility is perhaps the major focus of splinting the fingers, preventing loss of motion in the acute phases of healing and regaining motion in the presence of contracture. To achieve desirable outcomes, splint design must consider the pathology, the anatomy and the kinesiology of the hand, in addition to applying sound biomechanical principles. This chapter described a variety of splints that can be incorporated into a therapy programme that maximizes the functional potential of diseased or injured fingers.

References

Bell, J (1987) Serial static casting. In Fess EE, Philips CA (1987) *Hand Splinting: Principles and Methods* 2nd edn, St Louis: CV Mosby.

Boscheinen-Morrin, J, Davey, V, Conolly, WB (1992) *The Hand: Fundamentals of Therapy*, 2nd edn. Oxford: Butterworth Heinemann.

Bowers, WH (1987a) The anatomy of the interphalangeal joints. In: Bowers, WH (ed) *The Interphalangeal Joints*, pp. 1–20. Edinburgh: Churchill Livingstone.

Bowers, WH (1987b) Injuries and complications of injuries to the capsular structure of the interphalangeal joints. In: Bowers, WH (ed) *The Interphalangeal Joints*, pp. 56–76. Edinburgh: Churchill Livingstone.

Capner, N (1967) Lively splints. *Physiotherapy* 53: 371–374.

Colditz, JC (1995) Spring-wire extension splinting of the proximal interphalangeal joint. In: Hunter, JM, Makin, EJ, Callahan, AD (eds) *Rehabilitation of the Hand: Surgery and Therapy*, pp. 1617–1629. St Louis: Mosby.

De La Caffinière, J (1981) Topographic anatomy. In: Tubiana, R (ed) *The Hand*, Vol. I, pp. 265–273. Philadelphia: WB Saunders.

Dubousset, JF (1981) The digital joints. In: Tubiana R (ed) *The Hand, Vol I*, pp. 191–201. Philadelphia: WB Saunders.

Evans, RL (1995) An update of extensor tendon management. In: Hunter, JM, Makin, EJ, Callahan, AD (eds) *Rehabilitation of the Hand: Surgery and Therapy*, 4th edn, pp. 565–606. St Louis: Mosby.

Fess, E (1989) Convergence points of normal fingers in individual flexion and simultaneous flexion. *Journal of Hand Therapy* 2: 12–19.

Fess, EE, Philips, CA (1987) *Hand Splinting: Principles and Methods*, 2nd edn, St Louis: CV Mosby.

Minami, A, Kai-Nan, A, Cooney, W et al. (1985) Ligament stability of the MCP joint: a biomechanical study. *Journal of Hand Surgery* 10A: 255–260.

Rayan, G, Mullins, P (1987) Skin necrosis complicating mallet finger splinting and vascularity of the distal interphalangeal joint overlying skin. *Journal of Hand Surgery* 12A: 548–550.

Rennie, HJ (1996) Evaluation of the effectiveness of a metacarpophalangeal ulnar deviation orthosis. *Journal of Hand Therapy* 9: 371–377.

Stewart, K, van Strien, G (1995) Post operative management of flexor tendon injuries. In: Hunter, JM, Makin, EJ, Callahan, AD (eds) *Rehabilitation of the Hand: Surgery and Therapy*, 4th edn, pp. 433–462. St Louis: Mosby.

Tubiana, R (1981) Architecture and functions of the hand. In: Tubiana, R (ed) *The Hand*, Vol. I, pp. 19–93. Philadelphia: WB Saunders.

Tubiana, R, Thomine, JM, Mackin, E (1996) *Examination of the Hand and Wrist*, 2nd edn. London: Martin Dunitz.

7

Splinting to Address the Thumb

Introduction

•

Anatomy

•

Splints Designed to Immobilize the Thumb

•

Splints Designed to Mobilize the Thumb

•

Splints Designed to Restrict Motion in the Thumb

•

Summary

.

Introduction

The position, orientation and motion of the thumb afford the human hand unique opportunities for function. Stability is essential for force transmission to objects during grip and pinch, whilst mobility is necessary to orientate the pulp of the thumb to the pulp of the fingers for fine object manipulation. Mobility may be sacrificed to achieve stability in functional use of the hand. Disruption of the joint surfaces and/or the ligamentous arrangement is commonly associated with rheumatoid and osteoarthritis. Altered muscle function is associated with paralysis or spasticity secondary to either peripheral or central nervous system dysfunction. Both joint and muscle integrity have a profound impact upon the thumb's contribution to function of the hand.

Splinting is used to provide stability to the thumb in the presence of subluxation and to position the thumb such that it can provide an effective opposition post in the presence of muscle imbalance. Splinting may also be used to position the thumb and prevent maceration of the skin seen in severe cases of neurological dysfunction.

Anatomy

The carpometacarpal (CMC) joint of the thumb is a complex joint with motion and stability determined by the shape of the articular joint surfaces, augmented by ligament tension, and intrinsic and extrinsic muscular activity. The compressive forces transmitted through the joint in occupational tasks is believed to be one reason osteoarthritis of the CMC joint is relatively common. As can be seen from close observation of the orientation of the thumb nail, the movements of flexion/extension, and a small range of abduction/adduction, occur without rotation of the metacarpal. To achieve opposition, the thumb must first abduct to position the metacarpal on the part of the articular surface of the trapezium where rotation occurs. Without rotation of the metacarpal, orientation of the thumb pad to the pad of the fingertips is not possible. Strong gross grip and pinch involve abduction and rotation of the thumb. Movement at the CMC joint of the thumb is a result of the combined action of the thumb muscles and the constraining influence of the ligaments (Zancolli *et al.*, 1987).

The condyloid shape of the metacarpophalangeal (MCP) joint, surrounded by strong collateral ligaments and the volar plate sesamoid bone complex, allows motion in flexion/extension with passive deviation. The collateral ligament of the MCP joint of the thumb has two components, one of which is always taut giving the joint stability in full range of motion (Figure 1; Tubiana *et al.*, 1996). The greater length of the ulnar collateral ligament allows some passive radial rotation essential in opposition. This ligament is more commonly injured than the radial ligament. The

normal range of motion is quite variable in this joint.

The interphalangeal (IP) joint is a trochlear articulation. The ligamentous capsular structures are reinforced by flexor pollicus longus (FPL) and extensor pollicus longus (EPL) tendons. Joint stability is more important than mobility. Hyperextension is common.

The MCP joint capsular and ligamentous arrangements are reinforced by the fibrous aponeurotic formation in the thumb index webspace. This attaches to bone, tendon sheath and skin. Contracture of this and other structures spanning the webspace is very common with oedema in the hand following trauma, or from immobilization secondary to muscle dysfunction.

The control of thumb position for function is achieved by the intrinsic muscles. These muscles are arranged in a fan shape around the metacarpal. The median nerve innervated muscles are responsible for movements of abduction and rotation

Figure 1   Medical aspect of the MCP joint of the thumb with the ulnar collateral ligament exposed. 1, First metacarpal; 2, 3, two parts of the ulnar collateral ligament; 4, EPL; 5, adductor pollicus; 6, first dorsal interosseous; 7, second metacarpal. Reproduced from Aubriot (1981, p. 184).

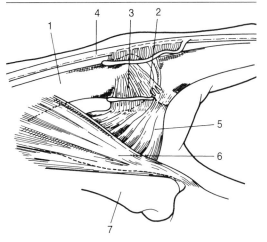

while the ulnar nerve innervated muscles produce adduction and flexion towards the fingers for grip and pinch. The radial nerve innervated extrinsic abductor and extensor muscles position the thumb away from the palm in preparation for grip and pinch. Splinting has an important role in sustaining functional use of the thumb in the presence of paralysis following injury to one or more of these nerves.

Splints Designed to Immobilize the Thumb

The thumb may be splinted in isolation or in combination with the wrist or the rest of the hand. Perhaps the most critical issue in design and fabrication of all thumb splints is the position in which the CMC joint is immobilized. This has implications for the maintenance of the webspace and rotation of the metacarpal to meet the functional requirements of the patient for grip and pinch.

A variety of splint designs are used to immobilize the thumb. In deciding which is the most appropriate design the two key issues for consideration are:

1. The pathology and the degree of immobilization required. Splints may address specific joint structures, or include more than one joint and the wrist if there is muscle or tendon involvement. It is not unusual that more extensive immobilization is undertaken in acute phases of healing, with reduction in size of the splint as greater mobility is allowed.
2. The patient's functional requirements. Function determines the forces that are transmitted through the thumb, and the requirement for skin friction and sensory input for object and tool manipulation.

IP Joint Immobilization Splints

Owing to the nature of the tissues in the thumb, a circumferential splint provides a more rigid means of immobilization (Figure 2). Cylindrical splints can be applied and removed easily, thereby avoiding problems with straps or tapes getting wet or needing to be replaced. However, sensory input to the pulp of the thumb is important for function and, therefore, modification of design will be necessary if grip and pinch are essential functional requirements. Plastic material is slippery and, therefore, prevents good purchase for pinch.

MCP Joint Immobilization Splints

When pathology is specific to the MCP joint, a decision has to be made as to the degree at which the splint will immobilize the metacarpal. Complete immobilization can only be achieved if the CMC joint is also immobilized, thereby prevent-

Figure 2   A thumb IP immobilization splint. The circumferential design has advantages for joint immobilization and dispersion of pressure; however, it limits the area available for sensory input during pinch.

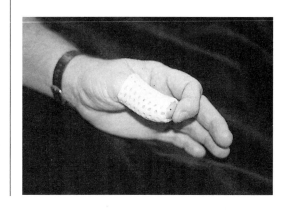

Figure 3 Thumb MCP joint immobilization splint. Stability for the thumb MCP joint is achieved without compromise to function of the thumb. The splint is secured with a Velcro® strap for normal function and taped into position whilst playing football.

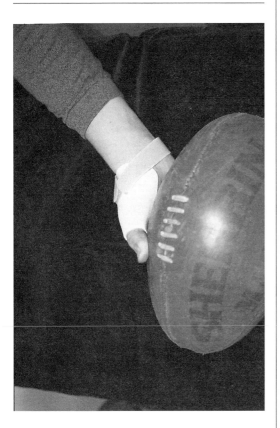

ing any rotation. A splint that protects structures around the MCP joint whilst still allowing rotation is designed to transmit much of the radial stress associated with pinch through the splint. Final stages of healing following ulnar collateral ligament injury of the MCP joint or arthritis are diagnoses commonly splinted in this manner (Figure 3).

THUMB MCP JOINT IMMOBILIZATION SPLINT

Procedure to take a pattern The easiest way to make this pattern is to wrap the plastic pattern material directly on to the hand with the distal edge just proximal to the IP joint. The pattern material should be approximately 15 cm square depending upon the size of the hand. Mark the following points referring to Figure 4.

1. Wrap the pattern material around the thumb and thenar eminence as indicated.
2. On the volar ulnar aspect, mark the circumference of the proximal phalanx from IP joint to proximal to the web at the MCP joint.
3. Mark the proximal end at the radial styloid at the wrist.
4. On the volar surface, outline the thenar eminence from MCP joint level to the wrist.
5. On the dorsal surface, outline the thumb through the middle of the webspace to the wrist.
6. A small extension is added to the circumference of the thumb to form a bond. The pattern should resemble the diagram in Figure 4b.
7. Cut out the pattern. Check for fit on the patient prior to transferring it to the splinting material. Splinting materials that have good mouldability are recommended for this splint.

Fabrication procedure

1. Position the arm on the table with the thumb in the required position. If there is a large difference between the circumference of the IP joint and the circumference of the phalanx, place some exercise putty around the proximal phalanx of the thumb.
2. Position the heated thermoplastic on the thumb as for the pattern, overlapping the area to be bonded. Mould the material ensuring the thenar eminence is well supported.
3. Slightly flare the proximal end ensuring it does not impede wrist motion.
4. When the material is cold, check the freedom

Figure 4   Thumb MCP joint immobilization splint pattern. Placement of pattern material is illustrated in (a), the shape of the completed pattern in (b) and radial view of the completed splint in (c).

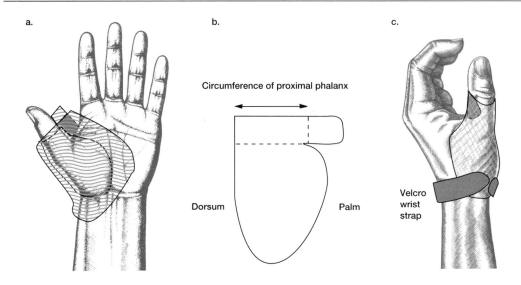

a.

b.

c.

Circumference of proximal phalanx

Dorsum

Palm

Velcro wrist strap

of IP motion. Mark any modifications required. Unseal the bond and remove.

5. Carefully reheat the two bond surfaces and reseal. Smooth the bond on the inside surface as well. Make any modifications required.

6. Attach the Velcro® strap.

Thumb MCP and CMC Immobilization Splints

Two designs for splints that immobilize the first metacarpal in relation to the finger metacarpals are discussed. Both immobilize the MCP and CMC joints whilst supporting the transverse arch of the hand. The hand-based design provides considerably more stability and provides circumferential contact around the length of the metacarpal (Figure 5). It is, therefore, used when the greatest stability is required as in the case of trauma, arthritis and neurological conditions with spasticity of adductor pollicus muscle. The spiral design maintains the thumb position in rela-

Figure 5   Thumb MCP and CMC immobilization splint. A hand-based thumb splint effectively immobilizes the thumb metacarpal and proximal phalanx in relation to the finger metacarpals. Wrist and thumb IP joint function is unrestricted.

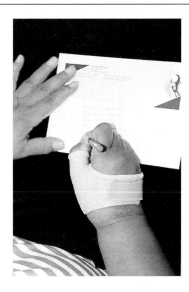

tion to the fingers, while maximizing the area of the palm available for sensory input and object contact. This design is commonly used to facilitate functional pinch grip in the presence of paralysis.

In peripheral nerve and spinal cord injuries, the forces transmitted through the thumb are not so great, therefore, this design is used more for positional control.

HAND-BASED THUMB MCP AND CMC IMMOBILIZATION SPLINT

Procedure to take a pattern You will need four measurements (see Figure 6). All measurements are taken from point 1 at the level of the distal palmar crease of the index metacarpal.

(a) Width of the hand just proximal to the MCP joints.
(b) Length of the thumb web – from point 1 to the IP joint crease of the thumb.

(c) Depth of hand through the thenar eminence.
(d) Circumference of the thumb at the IP joint plus 2 cm.

The dorsal and volar parts of this pattern are the same. In the centre of the pattern material, mark point 1 and draw a vertical and horizontal line through it. Mark the following points (see Figure 6).

1–2 Width of the hand (a).

1–3 Length of the thumb web (b).

1–4 Depth of the thumb through the thenar eminence (c).

From points 1, 2, 3 and 4 square across the vertical and horizontal lines, then mark in the following points.

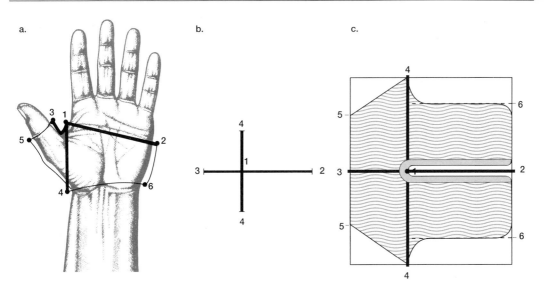

Figure 6   Thumb MCP and CMC immobilization splint pattern. The location of key markers are illustrated in (a), the linear measurements taken from point 1 are translated into a cross as in (b), which is the basis of the completed pattern in (c).

2–6 Length of fifth metacarpal proximal to the distal palmar crease plus 1 cm.

3–5 Half the circumference of the thumb plus 1 cm.

Fabrication procedure

1. To shape the pattern, draw a horizontal line from point 6 to intersect line 1–4. Curve corners where indicated.
2. Join points 4–5 with a diagonal line.
3. Cut out the pattern slashing down the vertical line 1–2. Transfer to the thermoplastic material.
4. To mould this splint, the thumb is placed in a position of opposition. If there is a large difference between the circumference of the IP joint and the circumference of the phalanx, place some exercise putty around the proximal phalanx of the thumb.
5. Remove the heated material from the water, then roll the edge the complete length of 1–2 away from the palm of the hand.
6. Place material on the patient's hand with length 1–3 through the thumb webspace.
7. Wrap the hand components across the metacarpals, proximal to the distal palmar crease, to slightly overlap and bond on the ulnar dorsal aspect of the little finger.
8. Wrap the components around the thumb pressing together into a flat seam the length 4–5.
9. Quickly mould the splint, ensuring correct position prior to cutting the bond 4–5 flush with the skin. This bond must be cut while the material is still warm.
10. Mould the splint ensuring good contour through the palm and on the dorsum of the hand.
11. When cold, unseal the bond on the ulnar

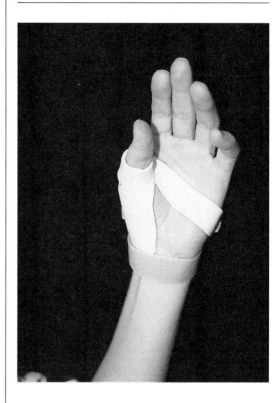

Figure 7 Spiral thumb immobilization splint. This splint immobilizes the thumb CMC and MCP joints with minimal impact to the palmar surface of the hand.

aspect and remove from the patient's hand. Trim the ulnar components.

12. Add an extra strip of material to reinforce the seam 4–5.
13. Roll the distal end of the thumb to allow clearance for the IP joint motion. Roll the component across the dorsal aspect of the hand so that the wrist motion is not impaired.
14. Attach Velcro® straps with adhesive-backed hook material on to the dorsum of hand.

SPIRAL THUMB (MCP AND CMC) IMMOBILIZATION SPLINT

Procedure to take a pattern Take a piece of pattern material approximately 25 cm × 15 cm, then:

Figure 8 Spiral thumb immobilization splint pattern. The pattern material (a) is wrapped around the hand. Markers determine the shape of final pattern (b).

a.

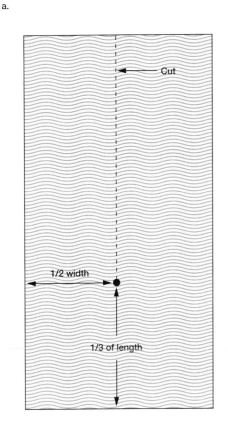

b.

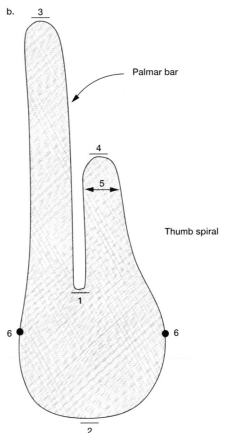

1. Mark point 1 at half the width and two-thirds the length of pattern. Cut the pattern though the length to this point as shown in Figure 8.

2. Place point 1 over the dorsum of the MCP joint and mark the wrist crease at the base of the thumb – point 2.

3. Wrap the palmar piece through the webspace across the palm and mark the length on the dorsal aspect of the ring finger.

4. Take the thumb piece and spiral around to encircle the proximal phalanx of the thumb. Mark this length.

5. The width of the thumb spiral is determined by the length of the proximal phalanx on the volar aspect of the thumb.

6. To determine the width of the thenar component, mark the thenar crease on the volar surface at MCP joint level and the middle of the webspace on the dorsum of the hand.

7. Cut out the pattern. Check the fit on the patient prior to transferring to the splinting material. Splinting materials that have strength are required for this splint. The thickness of material will determine the strength offered

by the splint – 1.6 mm for very young children to 3 mm for adults.

Fabrication procedure

1. To mould this splint, the thumb is placed in a position of opposition. Heat then cut out the pattern.
2. Apply the material to the hand orientating along the length of the metacarpal and the markers as identified in the pattern. Secure with a bandage if necessary. Ensure the thumb is in an appropriate position and the palmar bar is well contoured. Unless immobilization of the IP joint is required, splinting material should not impede movement.
3. The straps are attached with adhesive-backed Velcro®. An extra wrap of the strap around the wrist will increase anchorage of the splint.

Thumb MCP, CMC and Wrist Immobilization

Movement of the wrist and associated movement of the carpals does impact on pathology of the thumb. Post-reconstructive surgery or complex injuries of the CMC joint splints are required to immobilize the wrist as well as the thumb. To immobilize the thumb completely in relation to the rest of the hand, it is necessary to include all the metacarpals and the wrist. This is best achieved by a circumferential wrist immobilization splint with an extension to immobilize the CMC, MCP and, if necessary, the IP joint of the thumb. A description of the pattern and procedures for fabrication are found in Chapter 5, page 99.

RADIAL THUMB IMMOBILIZATION SPLINT

Where joint stability is not a concern, but pathology requires immobilization of the thumb and wrist, a radially based splint can be used (Figure 9). Tenosynovitis of the thumb extensor and abductor pollicus longus (APL) tendons (De-Quervain's tenosynovitis) is an example of pathology requiring this type of splint. Eliminating splinting material on the ulnar surface allows greater mobility of the hand and less impedance to sensation in functional grasp. This has an advantage to the patient who is required to undertake writing- or table-based activities.

Procedure to take a pattern The easiest way to make this pattern is to wrap the pattern material around the thumb and forearm so that the distal end is just proximal to the IP joint. The pattern material should be approximately 25 cm × 15 cm depending on the size of the hand.

Mark the following points (Figure 10).

1. The circumference of the proximal phalanx from IP joint to proximal to the web at the MCP joint.
2. Outline the thenar eminence on the volar surface from MCP joint level to the wrist.

Figure 9 Radial thumb wrist immobilization splint – radial view. The thumb is positioned so that opposition to the index and middle fingers is easily achieved.

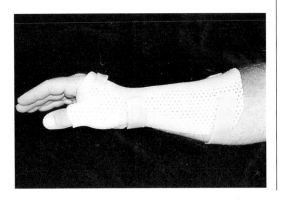

Figure 10   Radial thumb wrist immobilization splint. The pattern is illustrated in (a), with dorsal (b) and volar (c) views of the completed splint with straps *in situ.*

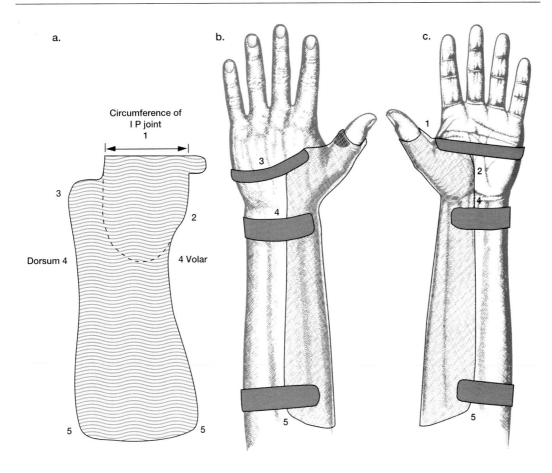

3. On the dorsum, the middle finger metacarpal at the level of the thumb MCP joint.

4. The wrist on the volar and dorsal surfaces in line with the middle finger metacarpal so that the width of the splint is half the circumference at the wrist.

5. Two-thirds the length of the forearm and the radial half of the circumference.

6. A small extension is added to the circumference of the thumb to form a bond. Connect marks on the thumb with those on the forearm so that the pattern resembles the diagram in Figure 10.

7. Check the fit on the patient and mark modifications. Adjust the pattern before transferring it to the splinting material.

Fabrication procedure

1. Position the thumb. Place some putty around the proximal phalanx of the thumb, if there is a large difference between the circumference of the IP joint and the circumference of the phalanx.

2. Position the heated thermoplastic on the thumb and forearm as for the pattern overlapping the bonded area. Mould the material, ensuring the thenar eminence and wrist are well contoured.

3. When the material is cold, check the freedom of the IP joint motion. Mark any modifications required. Unseal the bond and remove.

4. Carefully reheat the two bond surfaces and reseal them. Smooth the bond on the inside surface as well. Modify the areas marked.

6. Velcro® straps are applied to the proximal end and at the wrist. A narrow strap is applied around the hand. Place the adhesive Velcro® in the desired position and mark the correct location for the hook Velcro®.

Splints Designed to Mobilize the Thumb

Deficits in mobility of the thumb have a significant impact on the function of the hand. Serial splints are used to gain the range of motion in the webspace, while dynamic splints are used to address deficits in the MCP and IP joints.

Mobilizing Splints for the CMC Joint

Pathology affecting mobility of the CMC joint of the thumb, or soft tissues on the palmar or dorsal surfaces of the hand, will impact on the webspace between the first and second metacarpals. Mobility is influenced by the degree of abduction or extension, and flexion of the thumb and index MCP joints (Colditz, 1995). All splints designed to increase motion of the thumb joints compromise function during the period of wear.

Serial splints are the most effective means of addressing range of motion deficits in the webspace as intimate moulding increases the area of the first and second metacarpals over which force is applied. Long-standing contractures may require a series of splints. Time between remoulding to change position will depend on the compliance of tissues and their response to force. Once range of motion has plateaued, splinting can cease, if the patient is able to maintain the range by patterns of functional use. If function will not maintain gains, the patient may continue to wear the last splint at night.

A splint designed to increase passive range of motion in extension or abduction of the CMC joint must apply the force to both the thumb and index metacarpals and not the proximal phalanx (Figure 12). In the normal hand, the web extends past both the index and thumb MCP joints, therefore, these joints must be included if length is to be gained in the tissue. Webspace length is quite variable as indicated in Figure 11. Fear of shortening the collateral ligament of the index MCP joint (Phelps and Weeks, 1976) by maintaining it in an extended position in a mobilizing thumb splint is without basis unless the splint is on 24 hours per day, and active and passive movements of the joint are not undertaken.

Effectiveness of this splint is achieved by:

- Extended periods of wear at night or during times when functional use of the hand is not required.
- Application of force to the thumb metacarpal without stress to the ulnar collateral ligament of the MCP joint.
- Extending the splint to the distal end of the proximal phalanx of both the index finger and thumb.

Figure 11   Normal thumb index finger span. A normal span can vary greatly. To mobilize the region effectively, forces have to be applied to the metacarpal proximal to the MCP joint. The arrows indicate the appropriate location to avoid stress to the MCP joint capsular structures.

Figure 12   Hand-based thumb webspace splint. Dorsal radial view of the splint. The location of the strap is critical to achieve good anchorage and prevent distal migration.

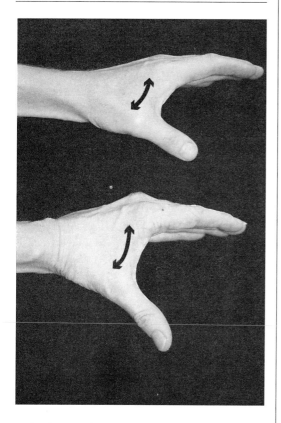

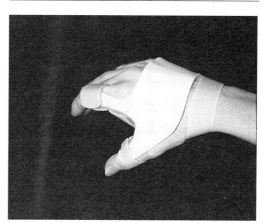

1   The length of the horizontal of the 'T' is the length of the webspace from the index finger PIP joint to the thumb IP joint.

2   The width of the horizontal of the 'T' is approximately two-thirds of the circumference of the thumb MCP joint.

3   The length of the vertical of the 'T' is determined by the distance from the volar surface of the thenar crease across the dorsum of the hand to the volar surface of the ring-finger metacarpal.

4   The width of the vertical of the 'T' is the length of the little finger metacarpal proximal to the distal palmar crease.

Fabrication procedure

1.   The splinting material is cut roughly to these dimensions, heated and moulded to the hand, ensuring excellent contour through the thumb index webspace. Pressure to abduct or extend the thumb (depending upon the objective) should be applied proximal to the MCP joints of the thumb and index finger.

- Anchoring the splint securely around the wrist to minimize distal migration.
- Selecting appropriate splinting material that provides good contour, and that can withstand pressure applied during fabrication and numerous remouldings.

CMC JOINT MOBILIZING SPLINT

Procedure to take a pattern A piece of thermoplastic pattern material is cut roughly in a very thick 'T' shape, and positioned through the webspace and across the dorsum of the hand (see Figure 13).

Figure 13 Pattern for hand-based thumb webspace splint. This serial static design uses measurements of the hand to shape the pattern (a). Dorsal (b) and volar (c) views of the completed splint illustrate one style of strapping.

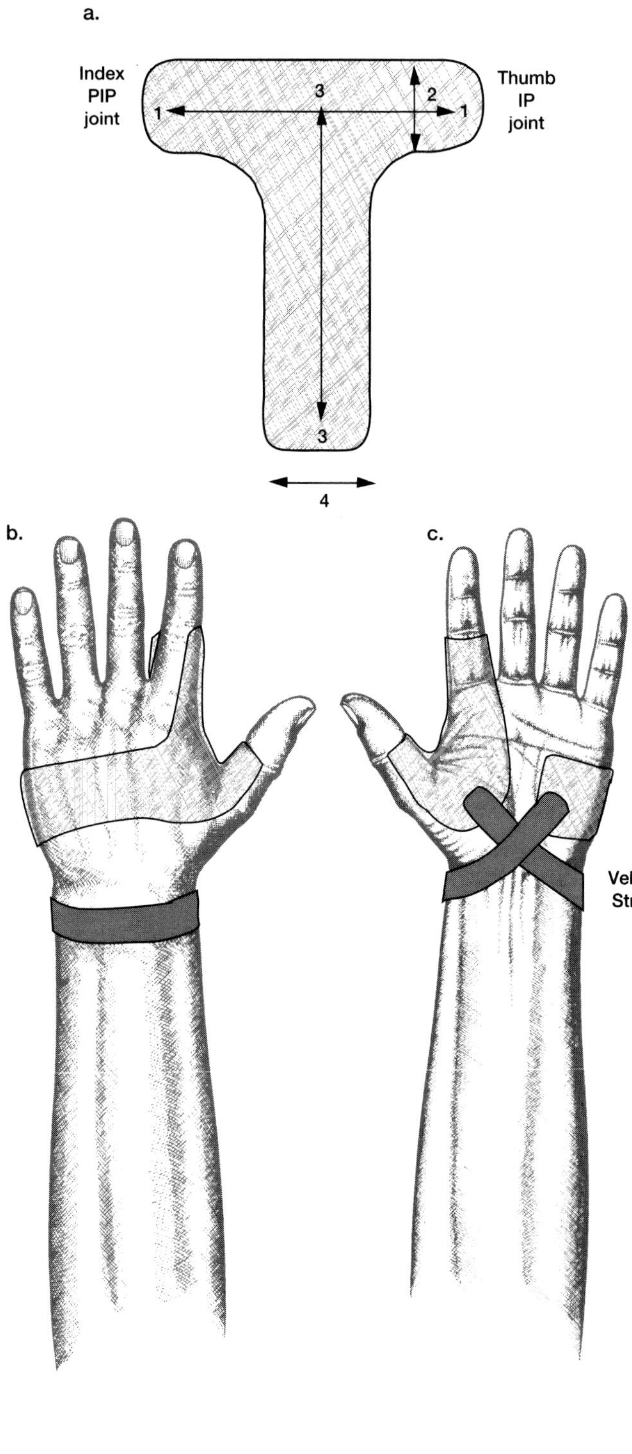

a.

Index PIP joint

3

2

Thumb IP joint

1

1

3

4

b.

c.

Velcro Strap

Figure 14   Hand-based thumb MCP and CMC splint. This design is used to mobilize the webspace used following surgical release. The splint was worn over a surgical wound with dressings secured by Coban (a), and subsequently a Lycra® pressure garment (c), so maxi-perforated splinting material was chosen to ensure some air could reach the wound.

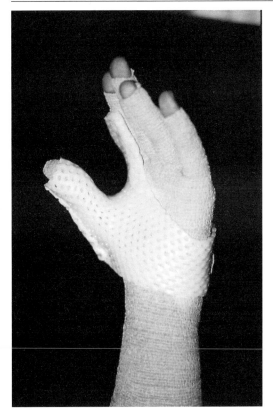

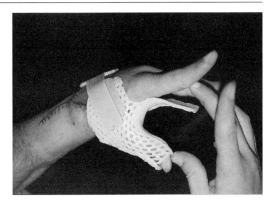

b

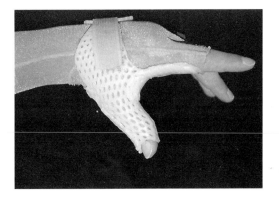

c

a

2. Once the material is cold, excess material is cut and edges smoothed.

3. The strapping must be spiralled around the wrist to prevent distal migration.

ALTERNATIVE PATTERN

For those patients who require greater anchorage, or for post-operative patients where straps could compromise venous and lymphatic drainage, the thumb MCP CMC joint immobilization splint is modified (Figure 14). The splint is fabricated in the usual way, then an additional piece of material is added to extend the webspace to the length of the proximal phalanx of the index finger.

Mobilizing Splints for MCP and IP Joints

Hand-based splints are recommended to address deficits in joint motion at the MCP and IP joints of the thumb (Figures 15–18). Care needs to be taken to ensure that rotational force is applied along the longitudinal axis of the thumb metacarpal to ensure no stress is applied to the collateral ligaments (Figure 16). The same principle is used

Figure 15 Dynamic flexion splint to address thumb MCP and IP joints. The deficit in thumb flexion is addressed by application of separate forces to mobilize the MCP and the IP joints.

Figure 17 Dynamic thumb mobilizing splint. Dynamic traction can be applied in the thumb to address one joint specifically by using an outrigger, as is the case in extension. A loop over the distal phalanx will address several joints in the direction of flexion to the palm. The wearing regime will determine the time the tissues spend at end range in each direction.

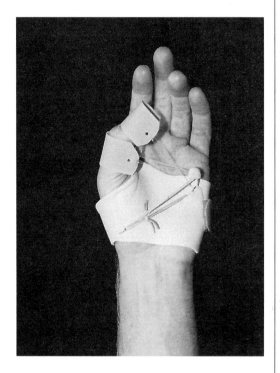

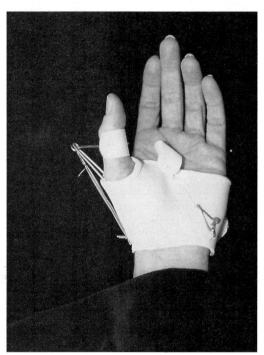

Figure 16 Appropriate application of multiple forces. Where several joints are mobilized in the one splint, it is important to ensure that the metacarpal is anchored and traction is applied along the longitudinal axis of the thumb as it is rotated towards the palm.

when applying traction to the IP joint. Deficits in extension of the MCP joint are often closely associated with contracture of the webspace, therefore, it may be necessary to combine gentle force to both the webspace and proximal phalanx.

The base splint to address a contracture of the MCP joint is the same irrespective of the deficit. Therefore, the splint must have components that traverse the palm and the dorsum of the hand both for stability of the metacarpal and anchorage of the traction. A thumb MCP and CMC joint immobilization pattern is recommended. It is cut

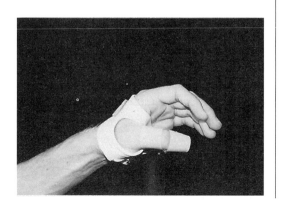

Figure 18 Dynamic thumb IP joint flexion splint. This series illustrates the change in anchorage required to ensure the direction of pull by the traction remains at 90° to the longitudinal axis of the distal phalanx as greater range is gained in the IP joint.

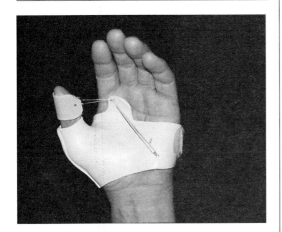

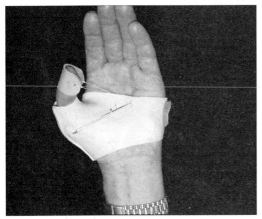

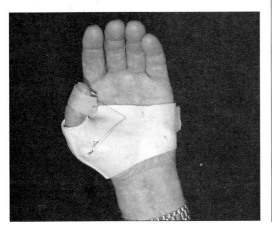

down to allow either IP or MCP motion. The procedure to determine the shape and location of the outrigger is described in Chapter 3, page 60.

If the ROM deficit is due to thumb extensor muscle tendon tightness impacting on several joints, then traction applied to the distal phalanx in the direction of the longitudinal axis of the thumb will rotate the thumb. Where there is little flexion, a loop over the nail will apply traction. As greater flexion is gained, adhesion of a hook or Velcro® to the nail is necessary to secure the loop.

Splints Designed to Restrict Motion in the Thumb

Splints that restrict motion in the thumb are used either to gain stability in the thumb for performance of functional tasks or to protect structures during healing.

Restriction during Wound Healing

There are many protocols described for the management of tendon repairs. From a splinting perspective, FPL is protected from full extension whilst EPL is protected from full flexion. Further information regarding protocols can be found in hand rehabilitation textbooks.

Splints that restrict flexion of the thumb are used following repairs to the EPL tendon. (Figure 19). The dorsal component extends from the MCP joint proximal whilst the volar component extends from the MCP distal. The wrist is immobilized in 30°–40° extension, CMC neutral to extension, MCP 5°–10° flexion and IP 0°. The degrees will be determined in consultation with the surgeon.

Figure 19 Dynamic EPL tendon repair splint. Following repair to the EPL tendon, restriction of flexion is achieved by the volar aspect of the splint distal to the MCP joint, whilst dynamic traction extends the thumb away from the volar block to facilitate tendon glide.

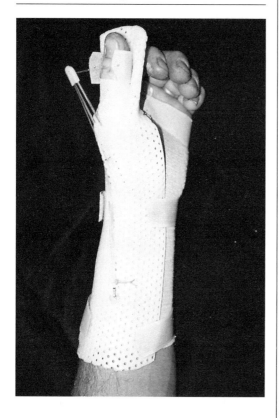

Procedure to take a pattern

The thumb is supported by the patient in a position of extension. The pattern material should be approximately 25 cm × 15 cm depending on the size of the hand. The pattern material is placed along the radial aspect of the hand and the following points are marked (see Figure 20a).

1 Tip of the thumb.
2 Half the circumference of the MCP joint on the medial and lateral aspects of the thumb. Add 1–2 cm to each side depending on size of the hand.
3 Half the circumference of the wrist on the volar and dorsal surfaces in line with the middle finger metacarpal.
4 The point at two-thirds of the length of the forearm and half the circumference on the volar and dorsal surfaces.
5 Cut between points 2 so that the thumb may be threaded through the hole. The components on the side of the thumb are folded volarly to reinforce the thumb component. Check the fit on the patient and mark any modifications. Adjust pattern prior to transferring to splinting material.

Fabrication procedure

1. Position the thumb and wrist with the required degrees of extension.
2. The heated thermoplastic is placed on the thumb threading the thumb through the hole created. Be careful not to make this bigger than the MCP joint circumference.
3. Fold volarly the extra width along the phalanges of the thumb. Mould the material ensuring the thenar eminence and wrist are well contoured.
4. Predetermined degrees of MCP and IP flexion are moulded into the volar block.
5. Attach the Velcro® straps.
6. Attach the outrigger and dynamic traction. (The procedure to determine the length and location of the outrigger and the length of the dynamic traction component is described on page 60.)

To restrict extension of the thumb, the splint is applied to the dorsal radial surface of the thumb, wrist and forearm. The pattern outlined in Figure 20 is modified. The material on the volar aspect of the phalanges of the thumb is applied to the dorsal surface (Figure 2d). The wrist is positioned in neutral and slight ulnar deviation, the CMC joint in neutral, the MCP

Figure 20 Thumb tendon repair splint pattern. The pattern to restrict extension or flexion of the thumb following tendon repair requires landmarks identified in (a). To restrict thumb flexion, it is placed through a hole at the level of the MCP joint as illustrated in (b).

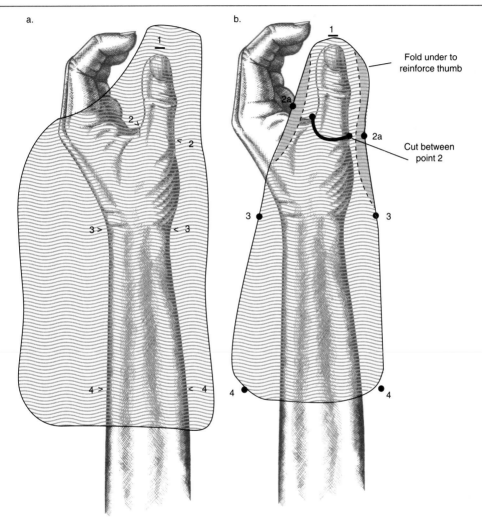

a.

b.

Fold under to reinforce thumb

Cut between point 2

and IP joints at 0° or according to the degree of extension allowed in the thumb joints. It is important that the passive flexion of all thumb joints is not restricted.

Restriction for Function

The nature of the skin through the webspace often means poor tolerance to the use of hard thermoplastic materials to position the thumb. Total immobilization of the thumb may also limit functional choices for hand use. Soft fabrics are incorporated into custom-made and prefabricated splints used to address the functional limitations of the thumb. In order to have an influence in controlling the thumb position, the fabric must have potential to resist the deforming forces created in the thumb during use.

Figure 21   Thumb flexor tendon repair splint. Restriction of thumb extension is achieved when the splinting material is placed on the dorsal surface of the wrist and thumb (left). Passive flexion of the IP and MCP joint should not be impeded by splinting material on the volar surface (right).

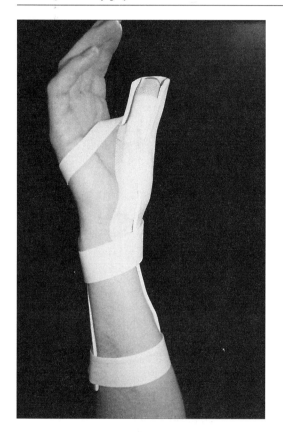
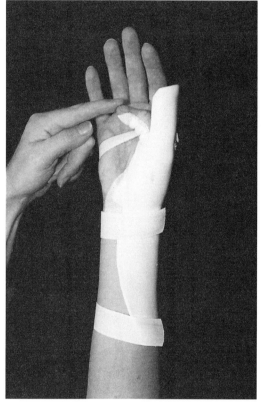

NEOPRENE THUMB SPLINT

This design, where the thumb is inserted into the hand base, allows more contour to the shape of the thumb, in addition to sustaining a rotated opposed position (Figure 22). Reinforcement can be added by directly adhering non-coated splinting materials to the neoprene. When used with young children with cerebral palsy, the bulk of the material is used to achieve the desired effect of abducting the thumb.

Procedure to take a pattern To make a pattern for this splint, a series of circumferential and length measurements are required. Place the hand on a flat surface and mark the following points (Figure 23).

1–2 Medial and lateral aspects of the hand just proximal to the heads of the finger metacarpals.

3 Thumb web just distal to the MCP joint.

4–5 Medial and lateral aspects of the wrist at proximal carpal level.

6 The index and middle finger web.

7 Tip of the middle finger.

Join points 1 and 2 (MCP line) and 4–5 (wrist line). Draw a line longitudinally through the finger from

Figure 22   Neoprene thumb splint. This splint provides some support to the thumb and provides warmth for this elderly lady with osteoarthritis.

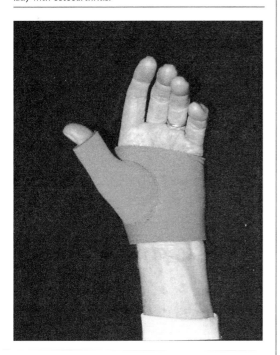

point 7 to intersect the wrist line. This line is the centre line of the pattern.

The following circumferences (indicated in circles in Figure 23b) and lengths determine the size of the thumb component and add to the dimensions in the initial pattern.

Circumferences:

1 Metacarpals at the level of MCP line.

2 Wrist.

5 Thumb at IP joint.

4 Thumb just distal to the MCP joint.

Lengths:

i   Proximal to index MCP joint to base of thumb web just proximal to the thumb MCP joint volar surface (1–3).

ii   Thumb MCP joint to IP joint .

iii Thumb MCP joint to the distal wrist crease.

iv   MCP line to wrist line at middle finger.

v   MCP line to wrist line ulnar side of little finger.

Fabrication procedure

1. Using the pattern in Figure 23c start at point 3 and outline the shape of the thenar eminence on the dorsal and volar surfaces. This slightly oval shape is cut out for the thenar eminence.

2. The thumb component is determined by the lengths between the IP and the MCP (ii) and the MCP to the wrist (iii). The width of the thumb component is determined by the circumference of the IP (5) and MCP joints (4).

3. The thumb component is folded in half and the two edges sewn together between the MCP and IP joints (i.e. 4 and 5).

4. Place this seam at point 3 on the hand piece. Ease the edge of the thumb component along the edge of the hole for the thenar eminence.

5. Sew two pieces together using a flat seam.

6. Closing for this splint is achieved by Velcro® hook and pile attached over the dorsal opening.

COMMERCIAL CUSTOMIZED AND PREFABRICATED THUMB SPLINTS

There are a number of brands of prefabricated thumb splints. They are made from a wide variety of materials including thermoplastic, elastomeric materials, neoprene and leather. They are secured by Velcro® tabs, with reinforcement for positioning or stability offered by metal or moulded thermoplastic components. The majority of brands are available in four or five sizes. The problems of fit may be compounded by the unusual shape of the thumb in cases where arthritis has destroyed joint integrity. Individual moulding of components, as is possible with some of the brands (Rehband®), increases the potential to fit the splint accurately and, therefore, meet the

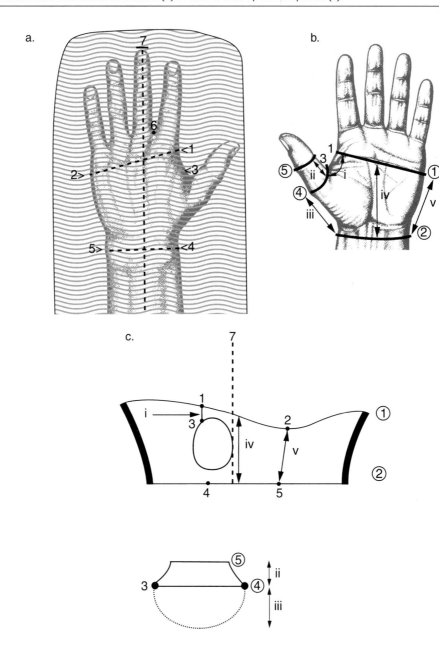

Figure 23 Neoprene thumb splint pattern. The basic shape of the pattern is made using landmarks identified in (a). The length and circumferential measurements identified in (b) are used to draw up the final pattern (c).

Figure 24   Commercially manufactured splints. Numerous brands are available. Rehband® short and long versions of thumb CMC MCP support are illustrated on the left and middle, with a Second Skin custom-made splint on the right.

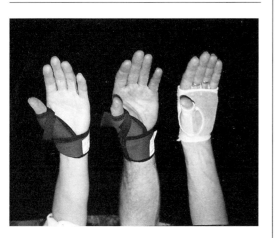

desired objective. Customized thumb splints made of Lycra® and leather allow unique designs to be created to meet the patient's specific requirements.

Summary

The function of the hand is dependent on a stable sensate thumb. Stability, essential for effective force transmission in the majority of grips and all pinches, can be achieved through splints incorporating joints of the thumb and, if necessary, the wrist. Deficits in active and passive range of motion, particularly as they affect the webspace, can severely compromise the ability to position the thumb for opposition to the fingers. Addressing these deficits via splinting demands an understanding of the unique architecture of the thumb, along with careful application of biomechanical principles in splint design and fabrication.

References

Aubriot, JH (1981) The metacarphophalangeal joint of the thumb. In: Tubiana, R. *The Hand*, Vol. 1, pp. 184–187. Philadelphia: WB Saunders.

Colditz, JC (1995) Anatomic considerations for splinting the thumb. In: Hunter, JM, Makin, EJ, Callahan, AD (eds) *Rehabilitation of the Hand: Surgery and Therapy*, pp. 1161–1172. St Louis: Mosby.

Phelps, PE, Weeks, PM (1976) Management of the thumb–index web space contracture. *American Journal of Occupational Therapy* **30**: 543–550.

Tubiana, R, Thomine, J, Makin, E (1996) *Examination of the Hand and Wrist*, 2nd edn. London: Martin Dunitz.

Zancolli, E (1979) *Structural and Dynamic Bases of Hand Surgery*, 2nd edn. Philadelphia: JB Lippincott Co.

Zancolli, EA, Ziadenberg, C, Zancolli, E (1987) Biomechanics of the trapeziometacarpal joint. *Clinical Orthopaedics and Related Research* **220**: 14–26.

8

Splinting and Casting in the Presence of Neurological Dysfunction

Introduction

This chapter is devoted to splinting clients with neurological dysfunction. The need for a specific chapter arises in part from the fact that expertise in splint design and fabrication is the domain of the hand therapist who rarely treats clients with neurological dysfunction, while therapists who have experience and expertise in addressing issues related to spasticity often do not have the same expertise in splint fabrication. The objective of this chapter is to attempt to marry these domains of practice.

In the presence of central nervous system dys-

function, the major motor problems are flaccidity and spasticity. Both impact upon the resting posture of the limb and the ability to move the limb through a full range of motion. When evident in association with either altered levels of consciousness, decreased sensibility and awareness of the effected limb, and lack of purposeful intent to move and use the limb, the consequences can be significant. These may be pain and oedema, joint subluxation, contracture of connective tissue, alteration in functional patterns of hand use, and breakdown of the skin as a result of pressure from approximation of body parts.

While there is discussion as to the practice of

splinting and casting clients with neurological dysfunction (Neuhaus *et al.*, 1981; Reid 1992), a significant body of empirical evidence supports the efficacy of this intervention. Splinting the client with neurological dysfunction is multifaceted and presents even the most competent splinter with some of their greatest technical challenges.

Literature Review

This brief literature review provides evidence of the historical process of splinting and casting in the presence of upper limb neurological dysfunction. As with all other areas of practice, where no one procedure is considered 'the right one', literature abounds with illustrations of practitioners' clinical experience of interventions they have used with success. This information provides the reader with building blocks for the evolution of more effective intervention in the future.

Splinting to Address Spasticity

The literature indicates essentially two approaches to the management of spasticity in the upper limb, emphasizing either biomechanical or neurophysiological neurodevelopmental perspectives. The biomechanical approach was the earliest form of treatment and adheres to principles of normal alignment, mobility and stability. Deformity and contracture are addressed by mechanical means. Splinting is considered an adjunct to positioning and exercise, with the rationale of preventing painful and otherwise troublesome deformities, rather than reducing spasticity.

With the advance in understanding of neurophysiology in the 1960s, the effectiveness of splinting was considered in the light of neurophysiological theories. Greater emphasis was given to the influence of sensory input in the design of upper limb

splints, along with the effect of sustained stretch and reflex inhibiting positions on the spastic muscle. In addressing the contraction associated with spasticity, splinting intervention used positioning to apply gentle continuous stretch to the spastic muscle at that range where the stretch reflex is initiated. This was at submaximal passive range of motion. It was proposed that positioning in this manner would reduce spasticity, by altering the threshold response to stretch of the muscle spindle and Golgi tendon organs in the antagonist and agonist muscles.

Much of the early research into spasticity reduction splinting for the wrist and hand addressed the surface of splint application (Kaplan, 1962; Zislis, 1964; Charait, 1968). Whilst the splint was used to apply sensory input selectively in relation to the spastic muscles, the influence of straps that secured the splint to the limb was not considered. Comparative studies by McPherson *et al.* (1982b) and Rose and Shah (1987) found the surface to which the splint was applied was not related to the reduction in tone seen in the wrist and finger flexors.

In addressing problems of spasticity in the elbow flexor musculature, the issue of the suface of splint application has not arisen. Circumferential designs are used in casts and splints, dynamic Lycra® splints (Blair *et al.*, 1995) and the soft foam circumferential splint (Wallen and O'Flaherty, 1991). Changes seen in resistance to passive stretch and range of motion are attributed to the inhibitory effects of circumferential contact and neutral warmth (Wallen and O'Flaherty, 1991).

Reflex-inhibiting devices such as the firm cone described by Rood (1954), Dayhoff (1975) and Jamison and Dayhoff (1980), and the position of finger abduction described by Bobath (1978), Doubilet and Polkow (1977), and Snook (1979) have been incorporated into splint designs. Designs for 'ball splints' and wrist splints incorporating cones found in the splinting catalogues (Smith and Nephew Roylan, 1995) have no publications to substantiate their clinical use.

Casting in the Presence of Spasticity

Much of the research on casting in the presence of spasticity is undertaken in single-case study design. Two groups of studies are seen – those that apply a series of circumferential casts worn for 24 hours per day for periods of up to 4 weeks, and those in which casts are bivalved and worn for periods of 3–5 hours per day for many months.

Casting has both biomechanical and neurophysiological effects. Biomechanical effects relate to changes in the length of muscle and connective tissues. Tardieu and Tardieu (1987) propose that muscle contracture seen in persons with spasticity is in part normal adaptation of muscle length in response to abnormal conditions. Histological changes in muscles in response to being maintained in a shortened position can be reversed by casting. The increase in passive range of motion (ROM) seen on removal of a cast results from the lengthening of connective tissue elements, along with addition of sarcomeres to the muscle fibre (Tabary et al., 1972). This results in a shift of the length tension curve, so that resistance met during stretching is less at a given angle. Loss of ROM after not wearing the cast or splint is due to reaccommodation of the muscle to the shorter length by the loss of sarcomeres. Thus, the objective of casting intervention in the presence of contracture is to achieve and sustain the appropriate length of the muscle and associated connective tissues. Casts applied by Freehafer (1977, 1978), King (1982) and Steer (1989) to elbow flexion contractures for 24 hours per day over several weeks resulted in significant gains in ROM. Decreased spasticity and increased control of movement were also noted (Tona and Schneck, 1993). Casts applied for periods between 3 and 5 hours per day over many months, maintained passive ROM in studies by Smith and Harris (1985), Cruikshank and O'Neill (1990) and Law et al. (1991).

The exact neurophysiological effects of casting on spasticity are undefined. It is proposed that inhibition results from decreased sensory input from cutaneous and muscle receptors during the period of immobilization. Application of gentle continuous stretch to the spastic muscle at submaximal passive ROM is seen to reduce spasticity by altering the threshold response to stretch of the muscle spindle and Golgi tendon organs in the antagonist and agonist muscles. The effects of neutral warmth and circumferential contact are also thought to contribute to modification of spasticity.

Splinting for Function in the Presence of Spasticity

Modification of spasticity and contracture offers the potential to improve voluntary motor functions submerged by the hyper-reflexia, dystonia and/or reduced joint mobility (Doubilet and Polkow, 1977). While it is assumed that, with improved joint mechanics, antagonists may be strengthened sufficiently to overcome increased muscle tone, the outcome in functional terms is rarely clearly defined.

The paucity of literature pertaining to the use of splints to facilitate functional use of the hand in the presence of neurological dysfunction is perhaps a reflection of the difficulties of research in this area rather than a window into the reality of splinting practice. Descriptions of splints in the literature are generally supported by single case studies. These include the orthokinetic cuff (Whelan, 1964; Neeman and Neeman, 1992), wrist splints with reflex-inhibiting components (MacKinnon et al., 1975; Woodson, 1988), a neoprene splint to position the thumb in abduction and the forearm in supination (Casey and Kratz, 1988), and splints to position the thumb in abduction (Landsmesser et al., 1955; Currie and Mendiola, 1987; Goodman and Bazyk, 1991).

Research findings from studies that investigated splints worn by children with cerebral palsy reveal trends toward more normal movement patterns and greater grasp skills (Exner and Bonder, 1983; Reid and Sochaniwskyj, 1992). However, differences are evident within the sample populations and in gains associated with splint wear. There was no significant relationship between splint type and change in hand function.

Where a variety of postures of the upper limb are required in the performance of functional tasks, rigid correction of deformity is not always compatible with function. Dynamic Lycra® splinting is a new innovation in splinting the client with neurological dysfunction. It was developed to overcome some of the functional limitations of thermoplastic splinting, particularly for children where the deficits in sensory input contributed to a modified motor output. Initial research into extensive body splinting using Lycra® has shown improved dynamic upper limb function with a reduction in involuntary movement (Blair et al., 1995). Improvement in patterns of movement is associated with a reduction in muscle tone. As previous researchers (Neeman and Neeman, 1992; Twist, 1985) have found, sustained cutaneous stimulation of the skin overlying spastic muscles results in relaxation of hypertonic musculature as evidenced by the limb assuming a more normal posture and disassociation from tonal patterns during intentional movement.

Summary

In the past 40 years, published studies that have addressed the issue of splinting and casting in the presence of spasticity have generally been of a qualitative nature. Variability is evident in sample size, the range of client groups in age, diagnosis and duration of symptoms; the types of splints and casts used; the wearing schedules; and the evaluation techniques used to determine the effectiveness of the intervention. The literature does not resolve issues pertaining the use of splinting and casting in clinical practice. However, when viewed alongside literature evaluating other forms of therapy, the deficits in this body of knowledge are not greater than that found for other therapeutic interventions used in the management of the upper limb for clients with neurological dysfunction.

Over time there is evidence of a gradual change in splinting and casting intervention, from that which specifically addresses spasticity and the consequences of deformity to that which focuses on dysfunction and meeting the client's objectives in occupational performance. The task of finding practical splinting solutions to complex and often technically difficult problems raised by the clients, continues to be the challenge confronted by therapists in neurological practice.

Assessment of the Upper Limb to Determine Appropriate Splinting Intervention

Assessment provides a baseline to determine whether alterations in the limb's posture, movement and function, are due to passage of time or rehabilitative techniques. Hand dysfunction should not be considered in isolation to the rest of the body. Retained primitive reflexes which influence head and limb position, and the stability and mobility of the pelvis, trunk and shoulder girdle, must be considered prior to determining specific functional deficits in the hand.

The next step is to identify the occupational performance objectives of the client and to analyse those aspects of musculoskeletal and neurological function that impair ability to participate in life tasks. Stresses associated with task performance must also be considered as they often result in movement patterns different to those seen in clinical testing. If the client does not have purposeful intent to use the limb, intervention focused on functional performance will not achieve any objective. Prevention of deformity for hygiene or pain relief then becomes the primary objective.

Lack of objective quantification of spasticity, associated patterns of movement and hand function are perhaps the major problems impeding advancement of clinical research in this area. An attempt should be made to define the nature of the resistance to lengthening prior to selection of a splinting programme. As spasticity has its greatest impact on intentional movement, observation of the limb during sleep may assist the therapist to determine if the problem is associated with con-traction of muscles or contracture of connective tissue.

Methods used to quantify spasticity in clinical practice remain primarily subjective. Clinical methods include measurement of:

1. The joint angle at which the stretch reflex is elicited on passive movement. This angle can be determined for elbow and wrist muscles.
2. The angle the joint assumes at rest.
3. The active and passive range of joint motion.
4. The functional performance of the upper extremity in tasks identified by the client as meaningful. The duration, quality of movement and method of completion of the task should be recorded on video for later comparison.
5. Recording surface electromyography (EMG) of the spastic muscle during muscle use, or the irradiation from the contralateral side during functional tasks (Kaplan, 1962; Zislis, 1964; Mathiowetz et al., 1983; Mills, 1984; Reid and Sochaniwskyj, 1992).
6. The extensibility and elasticity of the spastic muscle using mechanical devices (McPherson et al., 1982a, 1982b, 1985; Rose and Shah, 1987; Tona and Schneck, 1993).

Multidimensional assessment is required prior to determining appropriate splinting intervention. More objective measures are added to knowledge of changes in movement patterns in different postures, in activities requiring differing physical demands and cognitive skills, and at different times of the day and night. Without this information, splinting intervention may compromise function or alternatively be worn for no benefit.

Indications for Splinting and Casting Intervention

Modification of the Spasticity

In the presence of moderate to severe spasticity, modification of the stretch reflex is achieved by sustained uniform stretch having an impact on the muscle spindle. Splinting and inhibitory casting can place the elbow or wrist in submaximal passive ROM at the position of activation of the stretch reflex. Sustained cutaneous stimulation of the skin overlying spastic muscles is also thought to contribute to the decrease in spasticity seen during circumferential splinting, dynamic Lycra® splinting and casting.

Prevention of, or Modification to, Muscle or Joint Contracture

Where functional movement does not put the joint through a full range of motion, and daily passive range of movement or posturing does not adequately maintain range, splinting or casting may be indicated. Application of low-load prolonged stress to the contracted tissues at the end of their available range allows histological changes to occur in the tissues in response to the position imposed by the splint or cast. In the presence of spasticity, soft splinting materials are inappropriate as they have insufficient rigidity to sustain the joint at end range.

Maintenance of Integrity of Tissues

Where severe contracture and deformity have led to approximation of tissues, particularly in the elbow crease or the palm of the hand, intervention is essential to maintain extensibility of the tissues so that cleaning and hygiene are possible, integrity of the skin is maintained and infection prevented. Prevention of deformity and long-term maintenance are achieved by splinting.

Improvement in Function of the Limb

Splinting to address function may take two directions. In the first, intervention is designed to reduce spasticity and/or contracture. Intervention may compromise function whilst worn, but the gains subsequent to wear increase the potential for functional use of the limb. Secondly, splints are designed to meet specific functional objectives identified by the client and/or their carer, in conjunction with the therapist. Assessment will determine the requirements of the splint or splints, the design and the materials. If splinting allows success in performance of functional objectives, repetition of the task or activity will afford opportunities to improve strength, range of motion, coordination and skill.

Enhance Cosmesis

Limb posture and appearance are often an issue for adolescent and young adult clients. Modification of contracture and tone will affect appearance.

Long-term Management

Post-discharge from rehabilitation facilities or following extended holiday periods, it is not uncommon to see regression in clients with neurological dysfunction. Benefits gained from rigorous therapy programmes may have a longer duration if appropriate intervention is provided through splints or casts worn for specified periods during the day.

Contraindications and Precautions to Splinting and Casting Intervention

Splints and casts applied to the upper limb of clients with neurological dysfunction have the potential to injure tissue. The consequences of injury from incorrect or poorly fabricated splints or casts, or inadequately planned protocols may be permanent. Therapists should be mindful of the potential harm associated with these interventions, and put in place appropriate strategies for initial surveillance and ongoing review.

The precaution in splinting clients with neurological dysfunction relates to dissipation of pressure. Appropriate resolution of forces created between the client and the splint requires consideration of the dynamic aspects of spasticity and how it impacts on all features of the splint. Compromise of skin integrity and / or vascularity are potential risks.

Casting is contraindicated when continued monitoring is not possible and in the presence of conditions such as significant oedema, impaired circulation or heterotropic ossification. Precautions are required where there are unhealed wounds. External padding of the cast may be necessary for persons with behavioural or cognitive problems to ensure they do not injure themselves, or others, with the cast.

Dynamic Lycra® splints are circumferential in nature and made with fabric with an elastic component. Compromise of peripheral vascularity is a risk if the splint is not applied correctly, or mon-

itored for growth and change in dimension of the limb.

Patterns of Deformity and Intervention Options

The effects of neurological dysfunction are unique to each individual and tend to follow characteristic patterns of deformity. These are described as flexor or extensor patterns with shoulder retraction, depression and internal rotation, elbow flexion, forearm pronation, wrist flexion, thumb and finger adduction and flexion. Alternatively, the pattern may include shoulder retraction, depression and internal rotation, elbow extension, forearm pronation, wrist extension, thumb and finger adduction and flexion. In clients with cerebral palsy, scapular protraction and shoulder extension is also seen in association with the flexor pattern in the rest of the upper limb.

In the management of neurological dysfunction, identification of the pattern of altered muscle function is of vital importance in defining the objectives for splinting intervention. The information included in this section will identify patterns of deformity and discuss various options for splinting intervention. The patterns for splints are found in other chapters of this book.

Elbow and Forearm

The predominant pattern of spasticity at the elbow is flexion and forearm pronation. This pattern will limit reach and orientation of the hand in functional performance, and alter postural symmetry which has an impact on mobility (Figure 1). Severe flexion contractures of the elbow can also

Figure 1 The arm posture in the presence of increased tone in the upper limb. The inability to disassociate elbow flexion limits opportunities for incorporating the right hand into play activities.

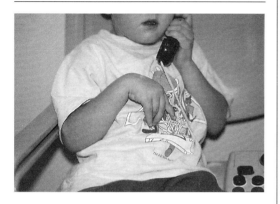

Figure 2 The arm posture whilst wearing a dynamic Lycra® extension supination arm sleeve. The arm posture has changed. When an arm sleeve is worn in association with a wrist gauntlet splint, greater opportunities for bilateral hand function exist.

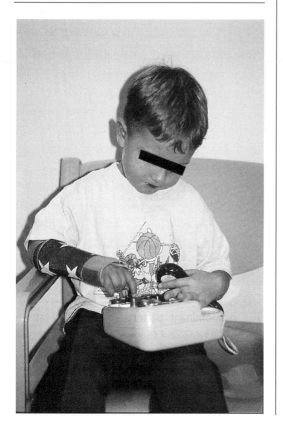

determine the ease for carers to position or dress the client. The pattern of elbow extension, forearm pronation creates fewer problems for care; however, it severely impedes any potential to use two hands in functional tasks of play or self-care.

RECOMMENDED SPLINTING INTERVENTION

In the presence of contracture, intervention should provide opportunities for the tissues to be held at end range, particularly when range can not be maintained by active functional patterns of motion (Figure 3). Casting over several weeks will maximize time tissues are held at end range, but is associated with the loss of limb function and normal deterioration associated with immobilization. When deciding to splint or cast the elbow to address contracture, a realistic end range of motion is determined by the functional objective(s) of the client, or the requirements of carers for passive motion in those persons dependent in personal care. Post-casting maintenance of range is achieved by bivalving the last cast or fabricating a thermoplastic splint (Figure 4).

Application of a soft foam splint to manage spasticity and contracture in the elbows of persons in acute phases following traumatic brain injury is described by Wallen and O'Flaherty (1991). The splint provides a continuous passive stretch through its tendency to return to its usual extended resting position. This property of the foam gives the splint a small dynamic action, as well as providing neutral warmth and circumferential contact. This type of splint also has application for management of elbow contraction/contracture in elderly clients who are confined to bed.

In facilitating functional use of the upper limb, rigid immobilization of the elbow is incompatible

Figure 3   A serial inhibitory elbow cast. Skin breakdown arose from the pressure of the approximation of tissues in the elbow in this client with dementia. Reduction in tone in the limb was evident whilst the cast was worn. A window at the elbow allowed access for wound care.

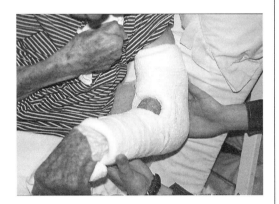

Figure 4   Elbow immobilization splint. The circumferential arm component on this splint increases anchorage and also decreases the potential to 'flex out' out of the splint.

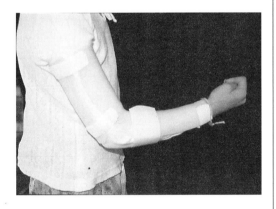

with function. Dynamic Lycra® arm sleeve splints use the inherent elastic properties of the Lycra® to facilitate either extension of the elbow and supination of the forearm (Figure 2), or flexion of the elbow and pronation of the forearm. Preliminary research using needle electromyography on normal subjects indicates a change in muscle patterns consistent with the direction of application of the splint (Gracies, et al. 1997)

Lycra® splints are custom made to the clients' requirements. Improvement is noted in the posture of the limb and the manner the limb is moved in performance of functional tasks. Thus, it is possible to address the elbow flexion forearm pronation tonal pattern that impedes reach without compromising the ability to bring the hand to the face for eating. Repetition facilitates re-education of the pattern of extension supination, with the potential to improve targeted function. Successes in performance of movements that facilitate function are repeated. This repetition affords opportunities to address strength, range of motion, coordination and skill, with patterns of deformity changing over time.

The prefabricated neoprene splint designed to supinate the forearm has distal anchorage on the thumb and a serial static strap to rotate the forearm. It is secured at the distal end of the arm. Flexibility of the elbow and wrist are possible. Casey and Kratz (1988) report success in facilitating supination with this type of splint in a single case study. The author's experience suggests this design is appropriate for clients who walk, who do not have a significant deformity of the wrist and who have functional extension of the arm.

Deformities of the Wrist, Fingers and Thumb

The wrist and hand present a complex interaction of intrinsic and extrinsic musculature in which spasticity dictates the predominant pattern of deformity, and ultimately the functional potential. In 1981, Zancolli and Zancolli described a surgical classification of spastic hand deformities in the wrist and fingers, while House et al. identified four patterns of deformity in the thumb. Building upon these classifications, modifications and additions focus on the functional deficits associated with paralysis and spasticity in the extrinsic and intrinsic musculature of the wrist, fingers and thumb.

In the following classification, static and dynamic aspects of deformity are considered. The dynamic aspect requires consideration as to which muscles have a primary role in the deformity or dysfunction evident. It is important to focus on the wrist first and determine whether the deformity arises from the wrist or the finger, or both the wrist and the finger musculature. This will assist in determining the appropriate therapeutic intervention of which splinting and/or casting may be options.

I. WRIST FLEXION THUMB ADDUCTION

Wrist and finger motion Mild spasticity in flexor carpi ulnaris (FCU) means function occurs with slight wrist flexion. However, strength in the wrist extensor muscles can overcome the spasticity. There is minimal evidence of spasticity in the finger musculature.

Thumb motion In a large number of cases, no deficit is seen in the thumb. The thumb deformity that is commonly associated with this wrist pattern is adduction of the thumb at the carpometacarpal (CMC) joint. Extension and abduction of the thumb are possible, but limited by a combination of contracture and contraction in the adductor pollicis muscle and first dorsal interosseius. Voluntary motion is still present in the thumb metacarpophalangeal (MCP) and interphalangeal (IP) joints.

Passive range Full passive ROM is available at all joints of the wrist and fingers. Contracture of

Figure 5 Pattern I: wrist flexion thumb adduction. The posture of wrist flexion of less that 20° seen on approach to objects.

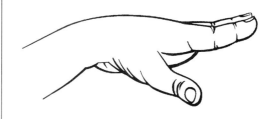

Figure 6 Pattern of thumb adduction at the CMC joint.

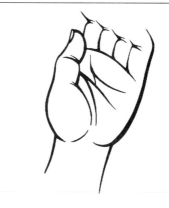

the thumb index finger webspace will reduce ROM.

Functional deficits This pattern creates no impediments to function of the hand. Approach to objects for reach and grasp is generally in wrist flexion, with a tendency for hyperextension at the finger MCP and proximal interphalangeal (PIP) joints. Finger flexion is well controlled and is associated with wrist extension. Hyperextension, seen at the PIP joints, results from wrist flexion increasing the distance the extensor digitorum communis (EDC) tendons traverse before inserting on the proximal end of the middle phalanx. Less shortening of EDC is required to effect extension at the MCP and PIP joints. Transmission of force through the fin-

Figure 7 Neoprene thumb splint. Neoprene allows some motion at the CMC joint with the 'bulk' of the material used to abduct the thumb. Bulk of material in the palm and failure to contour to the transverse palmar arch may impede grasp.

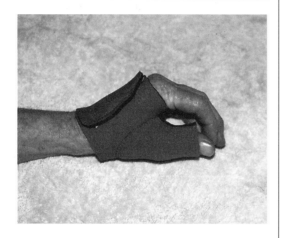

Figure 8 Spiral thumb CMC and MCP immobilization splint. This splint design maximizes the area of the palm available for sensory input. Material 1.6 mm thick was used for this child's splint.

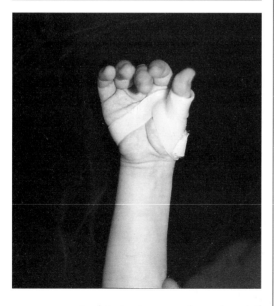

gers, as required in typing, may be reduced if hyperextension of the PIP joints is associated with PIP joint laxity. Thumb MCP joint hyperextension does tend to compensate for the defi-

cit in thumb abduction when grasping objects as large as the palm of the hand.

Recommended splinting intervention Intervention should be directed to specific functional objectives:

1. No intervention is necessary for the wrist as the gains from intervention would be outweighed by the loss of sensation and motion.
2. When the PIP joint deformity impacts on functional performance, small splints may be manufactured that restrict motion to the flexion arc by blocking hyperextension (see Figures 37 and 38 in Chapter 6).
3. If the deficit in active thumb abduction does not significantly impede function, decreased range of movement of the webspace may be addressed by a serial static splint worn at night. Functional use of the hand is not compromised.
4. Where thumb function is limited by inability to abduct for effective opposition, the splint chosen should abduct and rotate the metacarpal. Pattern and instructions for fabrication of thumb splints are found in Chapter 7. Splinting options are:
    (a) Custom-made thumb splints of either Lycra® or neoprene (Figure 7). Owing to the nature of these materials they allow movement, so are inappropriate if the adduction pattern is very strong or contracture of the webspace is significant. Designs that have the thumb component inserted into the palmar component of the splint are the most effective in positioning the thumb in abduction.
    (b) Thermoplastic splints to address the CMC and MCP joints and rigidly control the metacarpal. The CMC/MCP spiral immobilization splint design is recommended as

it covers a relatively small area of the palm, leaving wrist and finger function unimpeded (Figure 8).

2. MODERATE WRIST FLEXION, WITH ACTIVE WRIST AND FINGER EXTENSION

Wrist and finger motion Mild spasticity is located in FCU and flexor carpi radialis (FCR), with more severe spasticity in flexor digitorum profundus (FDP) and flexor digitorum superficialis (FDS). Strength in the wrist extensor muscles can overcome the resistance of spasticity in the wrist flexors as long as the fingers are flexed. Spasticity located in FDS and FDP muscles results in an inability to extend the fingers unless the wrist is flexed greater than 20°. Finger extension generally involves hyperextension of both the MCP and PIP joints. Spasticity located in the intrinsic hand musculature may impact on thumb and finger adduction.

Thumb motion On reach, the thumb may adopt a posture of adduction at the CMC joint, or CMC adduction with hyperextension of the MCP and IP joints. The thumb metacarpal is held in an adducted position by a combination of contracture and contraction in the adductor pollicus muscle and first dorsal interosseus. Action of extensor pollicus longus (EPL) and extensor pollicus brevis (EPB), acting across a hypermobile MCP joint, in the absence of flexor pollicus brevis (FPB) spasticity, creates the more distal deformity. Functionally, this deformity develops as extensors work to bring the thumb away from the palm of the hand for reach and grasp.

Passive range of motion No deficits are evident in the wrist musculature. Shortening may be demonstrated in FDP and FDS at the end range of finger extension when the wrist is also extended. Contracture of the index thumb webspace is generally present.

Functional deficits When approaching objects for grasp, the fingers are hyperextended at the MCP joints. The palm is not orientated toward the object for grip. The fingers can be posi-

Figure 9   Pattern 2: moderate wrist flexion, with active wrist and finger extension. Opening of the hand is associated with wrist flexion greater than 20°, closure of fingers is associated with wrist extension.

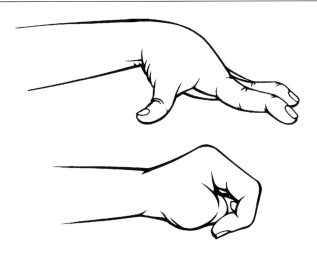

Figure 10   Pattern of thumb adduction at the CMC joint, and hyperextension at the MCP and IP joints.

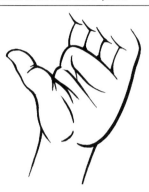

tioned over objects, a bar or handle, with increasing wrist extension evident as the fingers flex to grasp the object. With this pattern, the thumb is disadvantaged for effective opposition, particularly when associated with adduction at the CMC joint. Thus pulp to pulp pinch is generally unsuccessful unless the index finger is positioned in extension at the MCP and flexion at the PIP and DIP joints.

Functional requirements These clients require greater control of wrist motion – in flexion, so that the palm can be orientated towards the object on approach for grasp, and in extension, to give greater control to finger closure during grasp. Abduction of the thumb CMC joint and slight flexion of the MCP and IP joints increase the options for effective pinch.

Recommended splinting intervention Clients require more effective control of their wrist position. However, complete immobilization of the joint will only frustrate their attempts to use their hand as they have active wrist flexion and extension. The pattern of spasticity in FDS and FDP will determine the angle to which the wrist can be extended while still allowing finger extension.

Figure 11   Splinting intervention combining Lycra® and thermoplastic. The Lycra® wrist splint is combined with PIP extension-blocking splints to overcome a pattern of deformity exacerbated when undertaking this demanding fine motor and cognitive task.

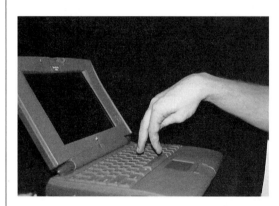

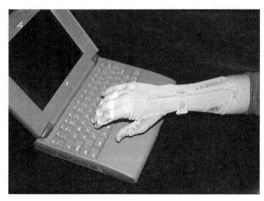

Immobilizing the wrist in a position approaching neutral may well compromise the ability to extend the fingers. Splinting options are:

1. Dynamic Lycra® splints have the flexibility to allow movement of the wrist through mid-range and, therefore, do not compromise finger function. Boning on the palmar surface will restrict maximal wrist flexion and extension. The thumb is rotated with lateral boning to provide stability for functional grip and pinch. The inclusion of a thermoplastic insert to abduct the thumb and stabilize the MCP joint

is warranted if boning does not modify the deformity.

2. Thermoplastic wrist immobilization splints made with the wrist at the degree of flexion that still allows active finger extension. Inclusion of components to immobilize the thumb will be determined by that deformity. The choice of a volar or dorsal design will be determined by the client's functional objectives.

3. Correction of the wrist position, and reduction of the distance over which the EDC tendons traverse at the wrist, will resolve much of the hyperextension deformity at the PIP joint. Splints to restrict the hyperextension are only necessary if the joints 'lock' in hyperextension, thus restricting co-ordinated flexion, or if the hypermobility of the joints compromise function.

4. Where the client is using his or her hand for functional tasks, other forms of splinting intervention should only be considered if there is evidence of contracture in FCU, FCR, FDP and FDS. The dorsal volar hand immobilization splint (Figure 13) can be used to address contracture during non-functional periods of the day, or at night.

3. MODERATE WRIST FLEXION, NO ACTIVE WRIST EXTENSION, WITH ACTIVE FINGER FLEXION AND EXTENSION

Location of spasticity Moderate spasticity is located in FCU and FCR, and the FDP and FDS. Strength in the extensor carpi radialis longus (ECRL) and brevis (ECRB) muscles is insufficient to overcome the resistance of spasticity in the wrist flexors. Wrist extension is very limited and may result from the action of EDC. Mid-range flexion of the fingers is possible; however, the position of wrist flexion dis-

Figure 12   Pattern 3: moderate wrist flexion, no active wrist extension with active finger flexion and extension. With no active wrist extension, active finger hyperextension occurs at the MCP joint on approach to objects. Full flexion of the fingers is compromised.

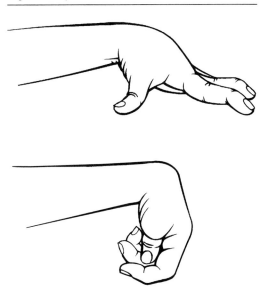

advantages the finger flexors as maximum muscle shortening is achieved before end joint range is reached. Hyperextension of the PIP joints is present.

Thumb motion The predominant posture of the thumb with this wrist pattern is adduction at the CMC joint and hyperextension of the MCP joint. As described in the previous classification, this deformity is a combination of contracture and contraction of intrinsic muscles acting on the CMC joint and extrinsic extensors acting across the MCP joint.

Passive range Significant deficits in extensibility are evident in the wrist flexor and extrinsic finger flexor musculature resulting in deficits in extension ROM. Shortening may also be present in EDC, limiting full passive finger flexion.

Spasticity located in FDS and FDP is evident on passive extension of the wrist.

Functional requirements These clients require greater extension of the wrist to enable the fingers to grasp objects towards the palm of the hand. Positioning of the thumb so that it can oppose the index finger will also increase options for effective grasp and pinch.

Recommended splinting intervention The objective of intervention may be to improve hand function, to prevent further wrist contracture for ease of management or to address pain in the wrist. With the predominance of spasticity in the wrist flexor musculature, the fingers cannot be tightly fisted and, therefore, there is rarely a risk of breakdown of skin in the palm of the hand. The associated deformity in the thumb will determine limitations seen in the webspace and range of motion.

Options for intervention are:

1. If spasticity is not evident during sleep, splints worn at this time can address contracture. The dorsal volar hand immobilization design is recommended (Figure 13).
2. Serial casting can be used to address contracture in the wrist flexors and extrinsic finger flexors. Casting is more effective than splinting to improve the range of motion as it maximizes the time tissues are held at end range. With greater length in these muscles, the wrist can approach a more neutral position and thus improve the biomechanical advantage to extrinsic finger flexor and extensor musculature during grasp. Gains from casting must be maintained with an ongoing splinting programme.
3. Functional splinting is used to gain a better

Figure 13 Dorsal volar hand splint. This splint can address wrist, finger and thumb position to influence spasticity or position at end range to address contracture. Radial and palmar views.

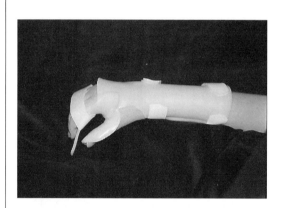

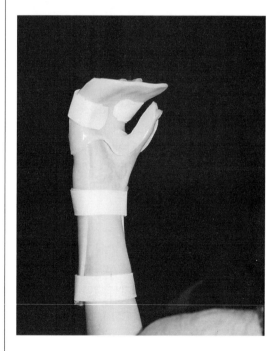

wrist position while not compromising the ability to extend the fingers during reach. The pattern of spasticity in FDS and FDP will determine the angle to which the wrist can be extended while still allowing finger extension.

Splints that address this deformity require rigid materials to hold the position.

(a) A dorsal wrist splint with a palmar component is recommended (Figure 14). This is not an easy position to splint therefore ensuring good contour and avoiding pressure on the dorsal aspect of the wrist is essential.

(b) Alternatively a dynamic Lycra® gauntlet splint, with significant reinforcing, is appropriate if rigid immobilization of the wrist compromises the ability to extend the fingers (Figure 15).

Figure 14 Severe flexion deformity of the wrist is exacerbated by functional use of the hand (top). Immobilizing the wrist in maximum passive extension with a dorsal wrist immobilization splint increases options for finger and thumb function (bottom). High-density foam inserted prior to fabrication of the splint modifies contour over the dorsum of the wrist. A customized lining 'sock' is worn under the splint.

4. Splinting options for the wrist should also incorporate components to address the thumb deformity. Abduction of the CMC joint, stabilization of the MCP joint in a few degrees of flexion, and prevention of hyperextension of the IP joint will position the thumb for effective opposition. To achieve this combination, rigid splinting components are used. Where functional wrist splinting is not an option as it would compromise finger function, splints designed to address the thumb deformity specifically can improve hand function. The thumb CMC/MCP immobilization splint design is recom-

Figure 15 Hand function is severely limited by spasticity in the wrist and extrinsic finger muscles (top). A Lycra® glove splint influences tone so that wrist and finger movement can achieve a more effective gross grasp (bottom).

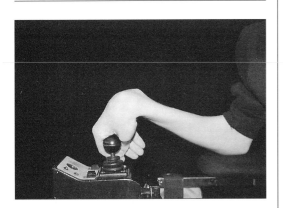

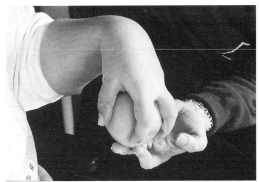

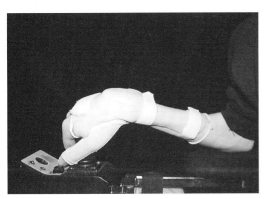

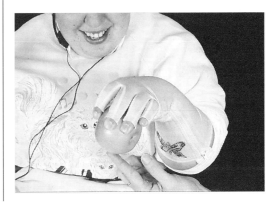

mended as it provides the necessary control to position joints.

4. WRIST EXTENSION WITH FINGER AND THUMB FLEXION AT THE MCP JOINTS

Location of spasticity Spasticity is primarily located in the wrist extensor muscles ECRL and ECRB. The other major component of this pattern is the intrinsic spasticity with flexion adduction at the MCP joints of both the fingers and thumb. A PIP joint hyperextension deformity may be associated with spasticity in the interossei muscles. With flexion of the MCP joints the intrinsic pull on the lateral bands of the extensor mechanism is facilitated across the dorsal aspect of the PIP joint.

Thumb motion The thumb metacarpal is held in an adducted position by contraction in the adductor pollicus muscle and first dorsal interosseus. The MCP joint is held in flexion by spasticity in

the FPB that does transmit some of its force to the IP joint via connections to the extensor tendon, thus maintaining it in extension. Contracture of the skin and connective tissue across the flexor surface of the MCP joint is common.

Wrist motion Active wrist motion is minimal with spasticity in the ECRL and ECRB sustaining the extended position. The strength of the wrist flexors in overcoming the resistance in the extensors determines the degree of active wrist motion.

Finger motion Contraction and contracture in the intrinsic finger musculature, combined with shortening in the EDC muscle tendon unit, limits motion into MCP extension, MCP abduction, and composite flexion at MCP, PIP and DIP joints when the wrist is in neutral. Where there is minimal contracture, effective finger motion is achieved with the wrist in neutral. Otherwise, MCP flexion and adduction predominate with finger motion primarily occurring at IP joints.

Figure 16   Pattern 4: wrist extension with finger and thumb flexion at the MCP joints. Wrist extension predominates with extension of fingers limited at the MCP joints. The thumb, flexed across the palm, compromises grasp.

Figure 17   Pattern of thumb adduction of the metacarpal combined with flexion of the proximal phalanx at the MCP joint. This pattern effectively eliminates any possibility of using the thumb for grasp or pinch.

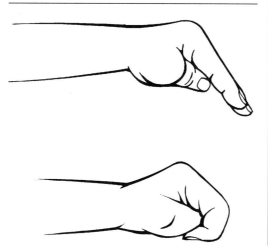

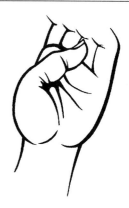

Passive range Deficits in range of motion are evident with contracture often present in the skin, wrist extensors, intrinsic finger musculature and EDC as seen by difficulty in achieving full passive flexion of the fingers with the wrist approaching neutral. Severe contracture of the thumb is common as it is trapped under the flexed fingers. Sustained pressure of fingers flexed against the palm of the hand can also result in hyperextension deformities of the DIP joints. Deficits are seen in extensibility of the skin and connective tissue over the dorsum of the wrist, the palm, and the webspace of the thumb and fingers.

Functional requirements These clients require the wrist to be positioned in a more neutral position to orientate the hand to approach objects and to allow motion of the fingers. In addition, the thumb must be extended out of the palm of the hand if any grasp is to be effective.

Recommended splinting intervention Without intervention, this pattern of deformity will lead to significant contractures of the thumb and finger MCP joints and ultimately a breakdown of skin in the thumb webspace and the palm of the hand. Hygiene is a primary concern. The objective of intervention may be to improve hand function, to prevent further wrist contracture for ease of management, or to prevent risk of maceration of skin in the palm of the hand.

Splinting options are:

1. Wrist immobilization splints made of thermoplastic materials are used to sustain a neutral wrist position. Designs must incorporate components on both volar and dorsal surfaces of the hand. The volar component incorporates the thumb in abduction and extension. This

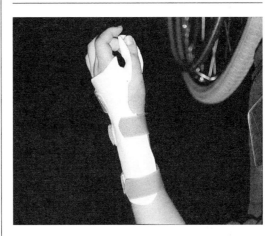

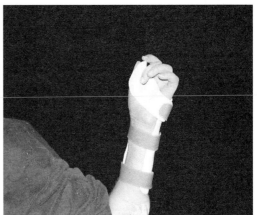

Figure 18   Dorsal wrist immobilization splint. The palmar bar of this splint is extended to place the thumb in a position that addresses the soft tissue contracture. Exposure of the pulp of the thumb would be appropriate if this client had an effective pinch.

splint can be used to address the contracture whilst also facilitating functional use of the fingers.

2. Serial static splinting is incorporated into the principles underlying application of wrist splints. Serial casting is an option should range of motion deteriorate despite splinting.

3. Protection of palmar skin is best achieved by addressing the wrist. Creating a space between the palm, the thumb and the fingers using soft

rolls or pads will address skin integrity. Numerous commercial styles and brands of 'palm protectors' are available. Where there is a hyperextension deformity of the DIP joints, rolls under the proximal phalanges are recommended as flat pads tend to exacerbate the hyperextension.

5. TOTALLY FISTED HAND WITH WRIST FLEXION OR WRIST EXTENSION

Location of spasticity The location of spasticity in the wrist musculature will determine the position of the wrist. Combined with spasticity in the extrinsic and intrinsic flexor musculature of the fingers and thumb, the potential exists for a severe deformity.

Thumb motion Severe adduction contracture of the thumb is always present. The posture of the rest of the thumb may vary depending on the contribution of other thumb muscles. Where FPL is involved, the thumb is flexed across the

palm and is trapped under the flexed fingers by a combination of contracture and contraction. Another common posture involves adduction of the metacarpal and flexion at the MCP joint against the radial side of the flexed index and middle fingers. Rotation often results from the sustained force applied to the fingers (Figure 21). Secondary connective tissue contracture compounds the problem.

Wrist motion No active motion is evident.

Finger motion Fingers are generally flexed at all joints with minimal active motion.

Passive range Significant deficits in end range motion result from contracture in muscles and connective tissue. Contracture is not always equal across the four fingers with the most severe deformity commonly seen in the ring finger. Constant approximation of tissues can lead to problems with skin integrity, nail care and hygiene.

Recommended splinting intervention The critical issue in this type of hand deformity is to maintain the range of motion so as to prevent fixed

Figure 20   Pattern of thumb adduction and total flexion. Contracture of soft tissue is commonly associated with this deformity.

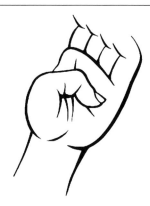

Figure 19   Pattern 5: totally fisted hand with either wrist flexion or wrist extension. A severe deformity where the fingers are tightly flexed over an adducted thumb.

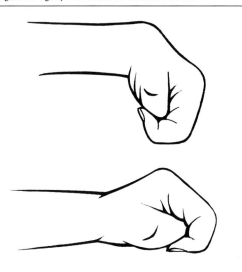

contractures, maceration, infection, and break-down of the skin on the palm and thumb. The objective is to stop approximation of the skin, to allow some air to circulate and tissues to dry. Splinting intervention must be sustained and reviewed on a regular basis.

Options for intervention are:

1. A spacer between the palm and fingers. Pre-fabricated palmar protectors and custom-made soft rolls can be compressed so they only create an interface between tissue layers. If placed between the fingertips and the palm, hyperex-tension of the DIP joint will be exacerbated. Ideally, spacers should be placed proximal to the distal phalanx to create gentle pressure on the proximal and middle phalanges, and not the distal phalanx.

2. To address the contracture, splinting interven-

tion must maintain length in the tissues. This can be achieved by adding firm components to rolls placed in the hand. It is suggested that the roll is the width of the palm of the hand with the circumference determined by the degree of contracture in the fingers and adduction of the thumb. Rolls made of splinting materials with large perforations, covered with an absor-bent fabric increase the potential for some air to circulate.

3. Where the wrist is sustained in extension, splinting to immobilize the wrist in a more neutral position will tend to open the fingers to allow separation of the tissues.

Splinting and Casting Procedures

Splinting clients with neurological conditions pre-sents therapists with some unique challenges that are not experienced in other areas of practice. Clients can not always position their limbs, or sustain a position that is ideal for the therapist. Spasticity will often increase owing to anxiety or excitement associated with the splinting proce-dure, on movement of the limb as the client attempts to assist, and in response to the tactile and temperature stimulus of the procedure. The therapist must not only control the splinting material, but also control the limb being splinted. Therefore, it is recommended the fabrication pro-cedure should be broken down into smaller com-ponents, and that material which has a memory is used. Attention should also be given to the envir-onment in order to reduce any factors that may increase spasticity during splint fabrication.

A thorough understanding of biomechanical principles, as outlined in Chapter 2, is critical in the design of splints for this client group. The

Figure 21 Adduction and flexion of the thumb has contributed to rotation of flexed fingers evident in the hand of a client with dementia. The wrist is in a position 40° extension.

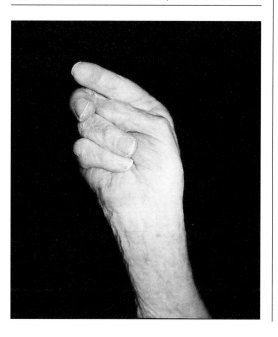

forces applied by the hand to the splint, and its various components, are significant. Thus reactive forces generated by the splint are equally great. Prior to designing a splint it is essential to analyse the normal forces generated by the hand, in addition to those generated by the spastic muscles. From this information, determine the direction, location and intensity of forces which will be created at the splint–hand interface when the splint is achieving its objective. Minimization of pressure is essential and is achieved by the strategic use of high-density foam padding and thick 'hand socks'.

Many of the thermoplastic splints used to immobilize or restrict joint function are described in the chapters on splinting the elbow, wrist, fingers and thumb. This section outlines some procedures that make it easier to splint the client with neurological dysfunction.

Dorsal Volar Hand Immobilization Splint Pattern

A combined dorsal volar splint (Figure 13) is recommended to address contracture and spasticity in both the wrist and fingers. This design is superior to the volar resting splint (Figure 6 in Chapter 5) because

- it uses an effective lever system to apply extension force to the wrist and fingers
- the pressure, resulting from force applied to position the wrist and counteract the force of the spastic muscles, is widely distributed across the dorsum of the wrist and the volar surface of the hand by well contoured splinting material
- it allows greater control over the wrist and hand so that it can be fabricated by one therapist

- it can be easily adjusted to accommodate increased extension of the wrist and fingers
- it can be applied independently by the client using one hand.

There are generally three issues to address – the wrist, the fingers, and the thumb. Prior to fabrication, determine the angles at which joints are to be splinted. Three millimetre non perforated Orfit or Aquaplast materials are used for this splint. Dense stockinette or woollen socks are used as a lining. They can be easily washed and replaced and are preferable to lining materials that are adhered to the splint. Allowance is made for the density of the lining material.

Procedure to take a pattern Mark the following points referring to Figure 22.

1. The length of the splint from wrist to proximal end is two-thirds the length of the forearm. This roughly equates to the length of the hand. Measure length using a tape and mark with a small dot.
2. Position the wrist at an angle close to the angle of the finished splint. Allow the fingers and thumb to remain flexed. Lie the pattern material over the dorsum of the hand and mark the points as illustrated in Figure 22a.
   1–2 Medial and lateral aspects of the hand just proximal to the heads of the finger metacarpals.
   3–4 Medial and lateral aspects of the hand at the thumb web level.
   5–6 Medial and lateral aspects of the wrist at mid-carpal level.
   7–8 Medial and lateral aspects of the forearm at the length previously determined.
   9 Index and middle finger web.

The width of the splint should be half the circum-

Figure 22   Pattern for dorsal volar hand splint.

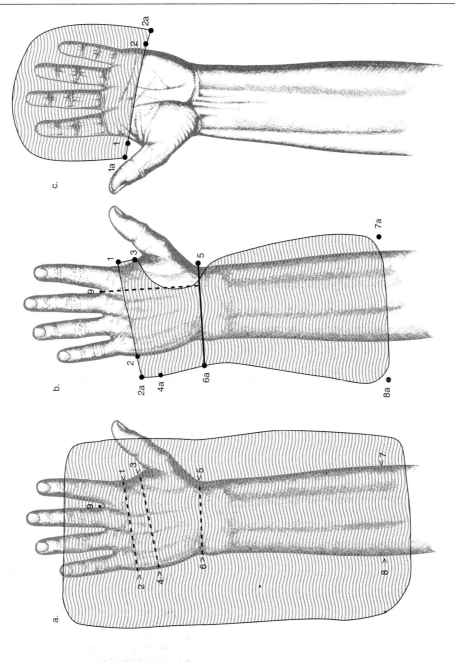

ference at the forearm and wrist. This can be determined by wrapping the pattern material around and marking the desired width at the forearm and wrist. These width points are indicated on the diagram as 2a, 4a, etc.

The volar finger component extends from the heads of metacarpals to the tips of the fingers. Flex the client's wrist to take the pattern. This will disadvantage the finger flexor muscles when contracting actively or in association with tone. Mark the medial and lateral aspects of the hand just proximal to the heads of the finger metacarpals as illustrated in Figure 22c. Add 1–1.5 cm to the length and width (radial and ulnar) of the finger component.

To shape the pattern:

1. Join points 1 and 2 (MCP line).
2. Join points 3–4 (thumb line).
3. Join points 5–6 (wrist line).
4. Draw a vertical line from point 9 to intersect the wrist line.
5. Starting at point 2a, draw a line around the forearm through points 4a, 6a and 8a, curve sharply around to 7a then up to 5. The curve through 7a should be shallow to ensure this aspect of the splint does not impede elbow flexion.
6. The line between 5 and 3 touches the vertical line 9 allowing clearance for the thumb.
7. Points 1 and 3 are joined.
8. Cut the two pattern pieces out. When fitted to the hand, the proximal edge of the palmar component is aligned to the thumb line of the dorsal component. Check for fit on the patient, prior to transferring it to the thermoplastic material.

The thumb position can have a significant influence on the tone in the fingers and the rest of the hand. An extra piece of splinting material is cut out. The dimensions are determined by the length of thumb, and the width of the thumb at the IP and MCP joint levels. For children under six, the thumb and the finger component can be combined in one piece of material.

Fabrication Procedure Moulding the splint follows the same sequence as taking a pattern:

1. Pad out any bony prominences on the dorsum of the wrist. If the wrist will be in greater than 40° of flexion, pressure will be exerted across the carpal bones, therefore, a piece of high-density foam can be used. Cut two pieces exactly the same size, with the adhesive backing on opposite sides. One is adhered to the client's wrist during moulding and the other will fill the deficit on the splint once moulded. If the wrist is in a more neutral or extended position, the padding is only required over the ulnar head and radial styloid. Intimate contouring of splinting material in the vicinity of the wrist is essential.
2. Place the heated material over the dorsum of the wrist and hand. Position the wrist while letting the fingers and thumb flex.
3. Prior to removing it from the hand, mark the location of the distal edge of the splint across the dorsum of the MCP joints. Remove it from the hand, reheat it and flare the edges.
4. Place the cooled forearm component on the dorsum of the hand, ensuring it is aligned to the marker. Flex the wrist until relaxation is evident in the fingers. The heated finger component is accurately positioned under the MCP joints and adhered to the forearm component on both radial and ulnar sides. Intimate moulding of the transverse palmar arch is crucial if this splint is to be comfortable.

5. Remould the finger component distal to the MCP joints to the predetermined angle of finger extension. This stage can be done without applying the splint to the client. Maintain the transverse and longitudinal arches.

6. In adult clients, where the circumference around the heads of the metacarpals is greater than the circumference just proximal to MCP joints, an opening may be required on one side of the splint for ease of access. Therefore, just before the material is completely cool, unstick the bond on the ulnar aspect of hand. The relative position of these two pieces of material is maintained by a Velcro® strap.

7. Apply straps at the proximal end of the splint and at the wrist, if the original pattern of tone was wrist extension. Finger straps applied to the proximal phalanx should have good contour.

8. Apply the splint and secure the straps.

9. The thumb component is adhered to the palmar surface of the finger component. It is important that the thumb piece is of sufficient width to mould intimately around the MCP joint to achieve a manipulatory force on the metacarpal in the desired position of abduction or extension of the thumb.

10. If necessary, a strap is applied to secure the thumb in the splint.

When fabricating splints in the presence of spasticity, determine the desired joint position prior to fabrication, then use the position of proximal and distal joints to decrease the effects of spasticity in the muscles traversing the joint to be splinted. Experiment with various limb postures to achieve the best position for the client and therapist. Initially therapists may require an additional person to position the limb with the second applying the material.

Dynamic Lycra® Splinting

Dynamic Lycra® splinting, an Australian innovation, offers some exciting new dimensions to the management of the upper limb in the presence of neurological dysfunction. Lycra® splints are custom made and designed to meet the client's functional objectives. Research has shown that Lycra® splinting has an impact on muscle physiology associated with abnormal tone such that changes are seen in the posture of the limb, the presence of tone and the agonist–antagonist balance in muscle action (Blair *et al.*, 1995).

To date, functional splinting has achieved its objectives by immobilization of the joint. It is proposed that Lycra® splinting achieves its objective by providing significant sensory input that has an impact on the underlying muscles, in addition to controlling joint motion. The principal advantage of Lycra® over other splinting materials is its ability to contour and conform to the changing shape of the limb during movement. The fabric allows movement but desires to return to its predetermined resting length and so will also facilitate movement according to the design principles incorporated into the splint. Movement of the limb, with a functional purpose, is therefore an essential requirement for prescription of this form of splinting.

Lycra® arm splints are designed to impact on the tonal pattern of the arm and forearm, facilitating active motion in patterns of elbow extension and forearm supination (Figure 23), or alternatively elbow flexion forearm pronation. Arm splints influence limb posture, and allow movement and weight bearing through a range of motion. Splints may be prescribed in isolation or in combination with hand splints. Splints that address the hand and wrist are designed to promote dynamic move-

Figure 23   Extension supination arm sleeve splint design. The splint extends from the axilla to the wrist. A forearm zipper increases ease of access.

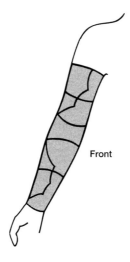
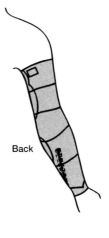

Front   Back

Figure 24   Lycra® gauntlet splint. Features of this splint include flexible plastic boning and leather on the palmar surface.

Figure 25   Lycra® glove splint. This splint extends from the tips of the fingers to two-thirds of the length of the forearm. Options for leather, boning, and single or dual zippers are available.

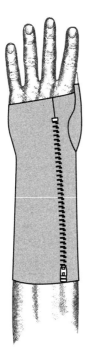
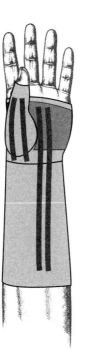
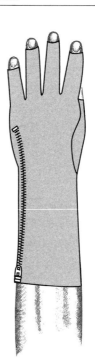
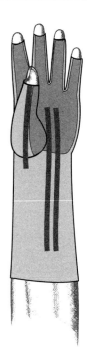

ment of the wrist, fingers and thumb to achieve effective pinch and grasp. Gauntlet splints (Figure 24) are prescribed when the spasticity influences the wrist position. With improved biomechanics for the extrinsic finger muscles, control in both flexion and extension is possible. In more severe patterns of deformity affecting wrist and finger musculature, a glove splint provides distal anchorage with greater sensory input to impact on involved musculature (Figure 25). However, difficulties associated with the application of a glove splint, and the fact that it is a more extensive intervention, reducing tactile sensation to the palmar surface of the hand and fingers, require consideration prior to prescription. Design features of gauntlet and glove splints incorporate flexible plastic boning moulded to support the wrist and thumb, leather palmar components to increase grip, and zippers for ease of application.

Client acceptance is high as many of the pressure problems associated with rigid splints and hard thermoplastic materials are eliminated. Incorporation of motifs and fashionable colours also add to compliance for children.

Casting procedure

Prior to initiating a casting programme for clients not within a hospital setting, commitment of carers to the programme is essential. The impact of the cast on posture and functional tasks such as showering, mobility, and dressing must be considered, and any problems resolved prior to initiating casting. It is also essential that the therapist and client are available for follow up for the duration of the programme. Holiday periods and summer months should be avoided. It is also suggested casts are not applied on Fridays unless weekend surveillance is possible.

Two persons are required. The person holding the limb is responsible for determining the angle the joint is to be cast whilst the other applies the cast. Prior to casting the angle at which each joint is to be immobilized must be determined. Fixing this angle by taping the goniometer provides an easy reference during the process.

Procedure to fabricate a rigid circular elbow wrist cast Stockinette, cast padding, thin wool felt, and plaster are required to manufacture this cast. Instructions are given for procedures for both the elbow and wrist components but they may be fabricated separately.

1. Measure the stockinette from axilla to finger tips (width of 7 cm for most adults and 5 cm for small adults and children). Cut a small hole for the thumb and apply to the limb. If the elbow is to be cast at greater than 45° flexion, slit the stockinette at the anterior elbow crease horizontally from one epicondyle to the other. Overlap the proximal and distal portions.

2. Cut the wool felt strips, 3 cm in width, to the following lengths:

   (a) The circumference of the arm just below axilla.

   (b) The posterior two-thirds of the elbow across the humeral epicondyles.

   (c) The circumference of the wrist just proximal to the ulna head.

   (d) Longitudinally down the posterior aspect of the arm, over the olecranon and down the shaft of the ulna.

   (e) Two strips are required for the thumb. The first piece is the length from the index finger PIP to the proximal wrist crease. Cut an oval hole in the middle and place it over the thumb at the level of the MCP joint. This lies at the volar surface of the index to thumb web and dorsal along the shaft of the first metacarpal. The second piece, the length from the index PIP joint across the webspace to the IP joint of the thumb, is threaded through the hole of the first and overlies it.

3. Tape the wool felt strips in place over the stockinette.

4. Apply cast padding in a circumferential manner in two parts: first to the arm, elbow and forearm, and then to the wrist and hand. Six to eight rolls of 7 cm padding are required depending on the size of the limb. Start at the proximal end of the arm placing the edge of the padding so that it overlaps half the width of the felt. Wrap it around twice before proceeding distally, overlapping the previous layer by half. 'Figure eight' around the elbow twice, overlapping the olecranon by 2 cm. Continue to wrap distally and end 2 cm proximal to the ulnar head. If the cast is to stop at the wrist, wrap padding twice overlapping half the felt.

5. Return to the proximal edge of the padding and apply a single wrap proximal to distal. Repeat. The padding should feel even throughout the length of the arm. Bulking or puckering of the padding may be smoothed out.

6. To incorporate the wrist, apply padding in a radial direction across the volar surface of the hand. Overlap the distal end of the forearm padding, and wrap it around the wrist to the base of the thumb MCP joint on the volar surface. Unroll a portion of padding about 30 cm long and split in half. One portion is wrapped around the hand while the other is spiralled around the thumb. Repeat this procedure twice so there are three layers of padding on the hand.

7. Apply the plaster using exactly the same procedure as the padding, i.e. in two sections. Begin at the proximal end of the arm 1.5 cm distal to the edge of the padding. Place small tucks in the plaster as necessary. At the end of each roll, moisten your hands and smooth the plaster in the direction wrap was applied. Repeat for a total of three layers.

8. After completing the arm, elbow and forearm, apply the plaster to the wrist and hand. When plastering through the webspace, pinch the plaster so that it lies in the trough formed by the padding. Do not plaster over the distal palmar crease to allow full movement of the MCP joints.

9. After completing the second layer, form the transverse palmar arch by applying gentle pressure with fingers on the volar surface, and the palm of hand on the dorsal surface. Hold it for 2–3 minutes until the plaster has set slightly before applying a third layer.

10. Finish the cast by turning the excess stockinette, felt and padding over the proximal and distal edges of the plaster and secure with a small strip of plaster bandage. Felt strips through the thumb webspace can be trimmed and then tucked in before securing stockinette with a small strip of plaster bandage.

11. Check to ensure that two fingers can fit snugly in at each end of the cast. The cast will take 24–48 hours to dry so it should be placed on a soft surface and pressure on the cast should be avoided.

After casting, the size, colour and temperature of the hand, and the capillary refill of the nail beds should be monitored. Staff and family members should be instructed how to monitor the cast and in the procedures to follow should emergency removal of the cast be necessary.

Casts may be worn for 4–10 days in a series over 3–4 weeks. Casts are removed with a plaster saw. On removal of the cast, the limb is re-evaluated, washed, gently mobilized and then recasted, if appropriate. To bivalve the last cast, saw the cast in half and carefully cut through the padding and lining. The stockinette is removed and a thin strip of felt taped over the edges of the plaster. New stockinette, and Velcro® straps are secured in place with thin strips of plaster. When applying a bivalved cast, it is important that the limb is positioned accurately in the cast to ensure no problems arise from pressure.

Wearing Schedule

One of the major drawbacks of the literature on splints designed to address spasticity is the poverty and variability of information provided about the wearing schedules in hours per day as well as total duration in days, months and even years. Studies by McPherson *et al.* (1982a) and Rose and Shah (1987) give indications for short-term outcomes (i.e. hours and weeks); however, further research is needed to ascertain appropriate wearing schedules in the long term. While patients in Brennan's (1959) and Kaplan's (1962) studies were splinted for many months, no indication is given for the reasons for discontinuing splinting.

A night-time wearing schedule has long been accepted practice and is often suggested in cases where splint application during the day is difficult (Snook, 1979). However, when clients exhibit very little spasticity in their limbs dur-

ing sleep, splints worn at this time will only position joints.

Immediately following splint or cast application, surveillance for at least 1 hour within the clinical setting is required to ensure no problems have arisen. Gradually increase the time of splint application, taking into consideration the client's tolerance. The bottom line for any splint-wearing schedule is compliance. Therefore, factors that increase compliance should be incorporated into the design and protocol.

Wearing Recommendations

1. Splints designed to address functional objectives should be worn during functional times only. Functional splints are never worn during periods of rest or sleep.

2. Splints designed to address spasticity are worn when spasticity has an impact on performance. There are no gains to be made by wearing splints at night if there is minimal evidence of spasticity during sleep.

3. In the presence of moderate to severe spasticity with associated contracture, experience suggests a period of splint wearing of between 4–6 hours per day is necessary to maintain extensibility of tissues in the long term. Splints should not compromise potential to use the affected hand.

4. Splints designed to address range of motion deficits may be worn at night when their impact on functional performance is minimal. In addition, this affords extended periods during which tissues can be maintained at end range. ROM gained by serial casting must be sustained by bivalve casts or splints until the risk of potential contracture is

diminished or active motion is sufficient to maintain joint motion.

5. Splints that have a preventative objective, whether that be to protect skin integrity or maintain length of tissue, need to be worn for as long as the risk exists. A lifetime of splint wearing is often a possibility.

Conclusion

Splinting and casting are valuable therapeutic interventions used to manage upper limb dysfunction in those persons with congenital or acquired neurological conditions. Published studies support the use of splinting and casting; however, they provide few practical guides to the therapist presented with the challenge of resolving upper limb dysfunction in this population. Information contained in this chapter on the common patterns of deformity, options for intervention using a variety of old and new designs and materials, and practical suggestions in design and fabrication, will assist those therapists prepared to undertake this challenging yet rewarding area of splinting.

References

Blair, E, Ballantyne, J, Horsman, S, et al. (1995) A study of the a dynamic proximal stability splint in the management of children with cerebral palsy. *Developmental Medicine and Child Neurology* 37: 544–554.

Bobath, B (1978) *Adult Hemiplegia: Evaluation and Treatment.* London: William Heinemann Medical Books.

Brennan, J (1959) Response to stretch of hypertonic muscle groups in hemiplegia. *British Medical Journal* 1: 1504–1507.

Casey, CA, Kratz, EJ (1988) Soft tissue splinting with neoprene: the thumb abduction supinator splint. *American Journal of Occupational Therapy* 42: 395–398.

Charait, SE (1968) A comparison of volar and dorsal splinting of the hemiplegic hand. *American Journal of Occupational Therapy* 22: 319–321.

Cruickshank, DA, O'Neill, DA (1990) Upper extremity inhibitive cast-

ing in a boy with spastic quadriplegia. *American Journal of Occupational Therapy* 44: 552–555.

Currie, DM, Mendiola, A (1987) Cortical thumb orthosis for children with cerebral palsy. *Archives of Physical Medicine and Rehabilitation* 68: 214–216.

Dayhoff, N (1975) Rethinking stroke. Soft or hard devices to position hands? *American Journal of Nursing* 75: 1142–1144.

Doubilet, L, Polkow, LW (1977) Theory and design of a finger abduction splint for the spastic hand. *American Journal of Occupational Therapy* 31: 320–322.

Exner, CE, Bonder, BR (1983) Comparative effects of three hand splints on bilateral hand use, grasp, and arm–hand posture in hemiplegic children: a pilot study. *Occupational Therapy Journal of Research* 3: 75–92

Freehafer, NA (1977/78) Flexion and supination deformities of the elbow in tetraplegia. *Paraplegia* 3: 221–225.

Goodman, G, Bazyk, S (1991) The effects of a short opponens splint on hand function in cerebral palsy: a single-subject study. *American Journal of Occupational Therapy* 45: 726–731.

Gracies, JM, Fitzpatrick, R, Wilson, L, Burke, D, Gandevia, S (1997) Lycra garments designed for patients with upper limb spasticity: mechanical effects in normal subjects. *Archives of Physical Medicine and Rehabilitation* in press.

House, JH, Gwathmey, FW, Fidler, MO (1981) A dynamic approach to the thumb in palm deformity in cerebral palsy. *Journal of Bone and Joint Surgery* 63A: 216–225.

Jamison, SL, Dayhoff, NE (1980) A hard hand-positioning device to decrease wrist and finger hypertonicity. *Nursing Research* 29: 285–289.

Kaplan, N (1962) Effect of splinting on reflex inhibition and sensorimotor stimulation in treatment of spasticity. *Archives of Physical Medicine and Rehabilitation* 43: 565–569.

King, T (1982) Plaster splinting as a means of reducing elbow flexor spasticity: a case study. *American Journal of Occupational Therapy* 36: 671–673.

Landsmesser, WE, McCrum, RC, Allen, JC (1955) The opponens spacer. *American Journal Of Occupational Therapy* 9: 112–114.

Law, M, Cadman, D, Rosenbaum, P, et al. (1991) Neurodevelopmental therapy and upper-extremity inhibitive casting for children with cerebral palsy. *Developmental Medicine and Child Neurology* 33: 379–387.

MacKinnon, J, Sanderson, E, Buchanan (1975) The MacKinnon Splint: a functional hand splint. *Canadian Journal of Occupational Therapy* 42: 157–158.

Mathiowetz, V, Bolding, DJ, Trombly, CA (1983) Immediate effects of positioning devices on normal and spastic hand measured by electromyography. *American Journal of Occupational Therapy* 37: 247–254.

McPherson, JJ, Kriemeyer, D, Alderks, M, et al. (1982a) A comparison of dorsal and volar resting splints in the reduction of hypertonus. *American Journal of Occupational Therapy* 36: 664–670.

McPherson, JJ, Kriemeyer, D, Gallagher, T, et al. (1982b) The reliability of spring weighted scales in assessing hypertonicity. *Occupational Therapy Journal of Research* 2: 118–119.

McPherson, JJ, Mathiowetz, V, Franczyck, N (1985) Muscle tone:

objective evaluation of the wrist joint. *Archives of Physical Medicine and Rehabilitation* **66**: 670–674.

Mills, V (1984) Electromyographic results of inhibitory splinting. *Physical Therapy* **64**: 190–193.

Neeman, RL, Neeman, M (1992) Rehabilitation of a post-stroke patient with upper extremity hemiparetic movement dysfunctions by orthokinetic orthoses. *Journal of Hand Therapy* **5**: 147–155.

Neuhaus, BE, Ascher, ER, Coulton, BA, *et al.* (1981) A survey of rationales for and against hand splinting in hemiplegia. *American Journal of Occupational Therapy* **35**: 83–90.

Reid, DT (1992) A survey of Canadian occupational therapists' use of hand splints for children with neurological dysfunction. *Canadian Journal of Occupational Therapy* **59**: 16–27.

Reid, DT, Sochaniwskyj, A (1992) Influences of a hand positioning device on upper extremity control of children with cerebral palsy. *International Journal of Rehabilitation Research* **15**: 15–29.

Rood, M (1954) Neurophysiological reactions as a basis for physical therapy. *Physical Therapy Review* **34**: 444–449.

Rose, V, Shah, S (1987) A comparative study on the immediate effects of hand orthoses on reduction of hypertonus. *Australian Occupational Therapy Journal* **34**: 59–64.

Smith, LH, Harris, SR (1985) Upper extremity inhibitive casting for the child with cerebral palsy. *Physical and Occupational Therapy in Paediatrics* **5**: 71–79.

Snook, JH (1979) Spasticity reduction splint. *American Journal of Occupational Therapy* **33**: 648–651.

Steer, V (1989) Upper limb serial casting of individuals with cerebral palsy – a preliminary report. *Australian Journal of Occupational Therapy* **36**: 69–77.

Tabary, JC, Tabary, C, Tardieu, C, *et al.* (1972) Physiological and structural changes in the cat's soleus muscle due to immobilization at different lengths by plaster casts. *Journal of Physiology* **224**: 231–244.

Tardieu, Y, Tardieu, C (1987) Cerebral palsy. Mechanical evaluation and conservative correction of limb joint contracture. *Clinical Orthopaedics and Related Research* **219**: 63–69.

Tona, JL, Schneck, CM (1993) The efficacy of upper extremity inhibitive casting: a single subject pilot study. *American Journal of Occupational Therapy* **47**: 901–910.

Twist, DJ (1985) Effects of a wrapping technique on passive range of motion in a spastic upper extremity. *Physical Therapy* **65**: 299–304.

Wallen, M, O'Flaherty, S (1991) The use of the soft splint in the management of spasticity of the upper limb. *Australian Journal of Occupational Therapy* **38**: 227–231.

Whelan, JK (1964) Effect of orthokinetics. *American Journal of Occupational Therapy* **18**: 141–143.

Woodson, A (1988) Proposal for splinting the adult hemiplegic hand to promote function. In Cromwell: FS, Bear-Lehman, J (eds) *Hand Rehabilitation in Occupational Therapy*, pp. 85–95. The Haworth Press.

Zancolli, EA, Zancolli, ER (1981) Surgical management of the hemiplegic spastic hand in cerebral palsy. *Surgical Clinics of North America* **61**: 395–406.

Zislis, JM (1964) Splinting of hand in a spastic hemiplegic patient. *Archives of Physical Medicine and Rehabilitation* **45**: 41–43.

9

Case Studies

Introduction

Planning and implementing intervention for upper limb dysfunction involves a process of synthesizing knowledge and skills in a logical and useful method. This chapter provides case studies to demonstrate the clinical reasoning process used by the authors to achieve this. Four case studies are discussed that identify the variety of management strategies used to impact on the problems identified by the therapist and patient. Emphasis is laid on the reasoning processes that contributed to the decisions made in relation to splinting intervention, drawing together the

information from all chapters presented in this book.

The clinical reasoning process is divided into three sections – the person, the problem and the process. The *person* identifies the 'who they are'. Sociometric history is gathered and critical factors identified. The social context within which the person functions is explored, focusing on family and other significant relationships. Responsibilities and support systems are identified. Activities of daily living (ADL),·and work and leisure status are determined. Financial or other burdens need to be recognized. This information provides the context within which the problem must be addressed.

The *problem* addresses the issues related to the pathology of the presenting issue. Information on the injury or disease and the tissues involved is determined by assessment and analysis of the pathology in relation to impairment, disability and handicap. The patient's occupational performance objectives are identified. The therapist's objectives are determined from analysis of the problems and, in an acute setting, usually related to impairment and disability. Once the problems and intervention objectives are identified, the process of designing the therapy action is commenced.

The *process* initially involves ascertaining critical issues that influence the therapy decisions. Considerations to be examined include the patient's pre-morbid function, the nature of the dysfunction and whether that has implications for a lifetime, and whether the focus of intervention should address management of wound healing processes or maximizing the functional capacity of the patient. Aspects of personal characteristics to be considered include the involvement of significant others as carers, responsibilities to be fulfilled, and issues of compliance and cognition. The vision for the future of the patient should be clear prior to designing and implementing the intervention. Therapy options are identified, and decisions made regarding the most appropriate choices and the mix of therapeutic activities to implement. This process can only be completed by utilizing the knowledge base provided in texts such as this to ensure all relevant confounding factors are acknowledged and addressed.

These case studies demonstrate the components of the clinical reasoning process specific to this text. The person is presented and problems are identified. Therapy options are listed and decisions regarding the splinting intervention are described. Alternatives for design, fabrication and implementation of the splinting programme are discussed. Pertinent occupational performance recommendations are discussed.

Case 1: Peter – Trauma

The Person

Peter is a 20-year-old man who lives in a large country town, 350 kilometres from a major city. Peter's fiancée and family are very supportive and live in the same town. Peter is an apprentice mechanic in a large mining company. He works on site for 2 weeks followed by 1 week off. Avocational interests revolve around sport.

The Problem

Peter was involved in a car accident, while on his way to work to an isolated mine site. The driver was not injured. Peter sustained an open comminuted fracture of the distal radius and ulna of his left non-dominant hand, and multiple lacerations from the windscreen glass over the entire length of the arm. He was admitted to a major hospital 18 hours after the injury. Following admission, an external fixation device was applied with two pins to the second metacarpal and two pins in the radius. Multiple fragments of glass were removed and large skin flaps approximated. Delayed medical attention resulted in significant infection in the many wounds in the arm. Peter was discharged home once infection was under control at 2 weeks. Intervention consisted of elevation of the arm, once daily passive movements and pain medication.

Seven weeks post-injury, the fracture and external fixation device were reviewed by the regional surgeon. He was dissatisfied with the lack of resolution of oedema and deficits in finger motion and referred Peter to a city hand clinic for intensive therapy.

On presentation to hand therapy there was significant pitting oedema throughout the hand, wrist and forearm. Extensor digitorum tendons were adhered over the dorsum of the hand with limited passive finger flexion. The thumb index webspace was contracted. Range of motion (ROM) at end range of elbow extension was limited; however, shoulder movements were full. Concerns were also expressed by Peter and his fiancée about the possible outcome and his potential to return to work.

PATIENT'S OBJECTIVES

Peter's goals included the resolution of pain and oedema, and the recovery of movement and strength in the wrist. He was highly motivated to return to his pre-injury occupation and sporting activities.

Critical issues affecting the clinical reasoning process In determining the course of therapeutic intervention consideration was given to:

1. The severity of the fractures, soft tissue injury and skin lesions, initial infection and current phase of wound healing.
2. The worker's compensation insurer's agreement to fund accommodation in the city for an intensive 3–4-week programme of hand therapy. Brief follow-up visits were also funded.
3. Education of Peter and his fiancée regarding the nature of the injury, the anatomy involved, the healing processes and the effects of therapeutic intervention. Peter was to be his own 'therapist'.
4. Peter's determination to return to his pre-

injury apprenticeship as soon as possible. This would demand a wrist that was stable, pain free and able to withstand the vocational demands of heavy mechanical work.

Problems, Therapy Intervention and Splinting Choice

Therapy was divided into three phases. These were prior to removal of external fixation, initial weeks after removal of fixation, and the final phase of strengthening and return to work.

PHASE I (WEEKS 7–12): PERIOD OF EXTERNAL FIXATION

Therapeutic interventions selected to address oedema in the hand and forearm were compression and retrograde massage. Coban was applied as a glove from the finger tips to the elbow. This modality was placed around the external fixator and changed daily following pin tract care. Gentle retrograde massage was undertaken by the therapist. Hands-on therapy afforded many opportunities to consider Peter's reaction to the injury, its legal implications, as well as to address fears of future function and vocational potential.

The pain experienced arose from the fracture site, from the drag of tissues on the pins of the external fixator and compression associated with oedema. Pain of myofascial origin was also evident in the scapulothoracic musculature. This was attributed to altered body mechanics associated with the weight of the external fixation and protective movements of the upper limb. Trigger point therapy and exercises resolved this problem quickly.

Significant oedema on the dorsum of the hand, and lack of movement of the fingers had resulted in a deficit in passive ROM in flexion of the metacarpophalangeal (MCP) joints, in addition to extrinsic extensor tendon unit tightness. On maximum flexion, the fingers were between 3 cm and 5 cm from the distal palmar crease. Resolution of finger ROM deficits was addressed with active and passive exercise and dynamic splinting. Gentle passive movements of individual fingers were undertaken following retrograde massage when the movement was not as restricted by oedema. Peter was instructed in slow passive movements of the MCP and interphalangeal (IP) joints. Composite movements of the digits and individual joints were undertaken to stretch both the intrinsic and extrinsic musculature and capsular structures. This also created glide of the finger extensor tendons individually as well as a group. Activity provided direction to active movements used to facilitate tendon glide.

The location of one pin site on the second metacarpal had significant implications to swelling and motion in the index thumb webspace. Active and passive motion of the thumb was undertaken; however, tolerance to any form of pressure in this region was negligible.

Splinting alternatives and rationale A splint was required to support the weight of the hand and decrease drag on the external fixator. Factors that were considered in selection of splint design were:

1. The presence of the external fixator, with potential to modify the splint for use once the fixator was removed.
2. Significant pitting oedema in the hand and forearm:
   (a) With reduction of oedema, remoulding of the splint would be required.
   (b) Uniform pressure the length of the forearm

was required to eliminate risks associated with straps.
3. The need for a base for the application of dynamic traction to address the deficits in ROM of the fingers.
4. Possible future splinting intervention:
   (a) The need for wrist support following removal of the fixator.
   (b) The deficit in wrist and forearm motion requiring some form of mobilizing splint.

A circumferential wrist immobilization splint was made as the design fulfilled the requirements (Figure 1). Orfit® Classic 2 mm micro-perforated splinting material was chosen as it has the required strength in a circumferential design, many small

Figure 1 Circumferential wrist immobilization splint. An advantageous design to accommodate an external fixator.

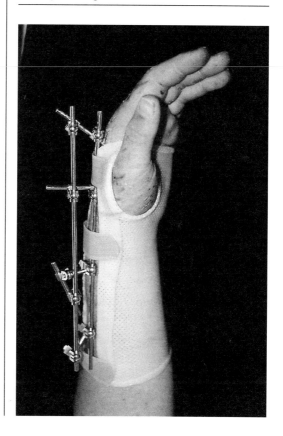

Figure 2   Dynamic traction applied to the middle, ring and little finger MCP joints to address deficit in passive ROM. Force was not applied to the index finger owing to pain associated with the external fixator.

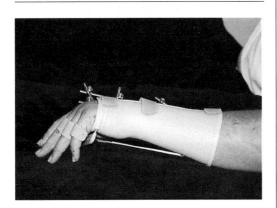

Figure 3   Dynamic MCP flexion traction applied via a removable outrigger.

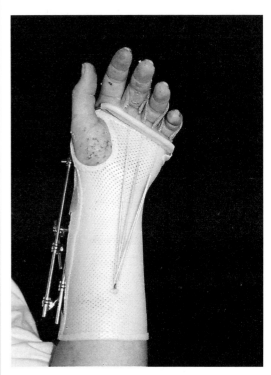

perforations to allow skin to breathe, properties which allow easy application to the limb without need for pressure for moulding and a memory to facilitate frequent remoulding.

A detachable outrigger was applied to the wrist splint so that traction could be applied intermittently (Figures 2 and 3). During other times, exercise and functional activities could be undertaken without impediment. Loops were initially positioned over the proximal phalanx of each finger to address the deficit in passive ROM at the MCP joint. Force was measured at 250 g at the anchorage point of the traction on the assumption that some of this would be lost in friction at the pulley of the outrigger. Once full ROM was possible at the MCP joints, the outrigger was modified so that traction was applied to the distal phalanx to address the tendon length across all three joints. The splint was worn at all times. The outrigger was attached for periods of 2 hours three times per day. This time was determined by tolerance and the opportunity to use the hand in functional activities. The outrigger was discarded after 18 days when the fingertips could touch the palm.

Active motion of the fingers was encouraged during performance of light functional tasks and during periods when the outrigger was not attached. A home programme was instigated with retrograde massage undertaken by Peter. Coban was applied by his fiancée, and active and passive finger and thumb motion combined with dynamic splinting. Peter went home after 3 weeks of therapy and returned immediately following removal of the external fixation device.

PHASE 2 (WEEKS 12–18): POST-REMOVAL OF EXTERNAL FIXATION

The 2 weeks of therapy immediately following removal of the fixation were primarily directed at regaining range of motion. Significant reduction was seen in oedema following the application of Coban; however, residual oedema was present. Multiple small scars the length of the arm from glass lacerations remained red and raised, and were hypertrophic. A custom-made Lycra® garment was applied from fingertip to axilla to address both oedema and scarring. Splints were remoulded to fit over the top of the garment, which was retensioned as oedema resolved. It was worn throughout the day and evening from the time of application with gradual weaning around 24 weeks. Whilst the garment did impact on the hypertrophic scars, Peter decided to discard the garment at this time, preferring to get back to work without any encumbrance. Appearance of the scars was not an issue.

Splinting alternatives and rationale The wrist immobilization splint was worn between exercise periods until strength in the wrist extensor musculature was sufficient to sustain the wrist position against gravity.

Regaining range of motion was the primary objective of intervention at this stage. Deficits were identified in the thumb index webspace, with wrist ROM 0°–11° extension, 0°–26° flexion, 0°–85° pronation and 0°–19° supination. The severity of the injury suggested that recovery of significant wrist motion was unrealistic. Peter determined that at least 30° in wrist flexion and extension, and 60° supination would be vocationally useful. Pain experienced at end range of motion and on force transmission through the wrist would ultimately determine the functional potential of the left upper limb.

The primary choice of intervention was a mobilizing splint as muscle strength was insufficient to achieve end range, and passive mobilization via continuous passive motion (CPM) machine was limited to periods of 45–60 minutes daily while able to attend therapy. Emphasis was placed on thumb extension, wrist extension and forearm supination as gains had implications to performance of functional and vocational tasks.

Serial static splinting was considered for the deficit in the index thumb webspace. As support was still required for the wrist, a hand-based splint was inappropriate. Therefore, the wrist was incorporated into the design (Figure 5 in Chapter 1). NCM Preferred was used as this splinting material allows intimate mould to ensure contour, and even pressure was applied in the end range position in both wrist and thumb extension. The material tolerated remoulding as the range of motion changed. This splint was worn at night as sleep afforded an extended period of time to address ROM deficits. It was discarded after 5 weeks when the thumb range of motion plateaued (Figure 4) and wrist strength was sufficient to maintain position.

As Peter was unavailable for intensive therapy, a dynamic splint was chosen to apply a gentle force for maximum time at end range. With his mechanical background, Peter understood the principles of applying dynamic traction and the therapist was confident he could modify the dynamic wrist splint outrigger as his range of wrist motion increased.

A dynamic splint was fabricated for the wrist (Figure 19 in Chapter 5). The two-piece design with a swivel hinge allowed for placement of outriggers in both flexion and extension. However, only the extension outrigger was used as gains in flexion were considered acceptable for function. Sansplint XR® (Polyflex®) was used for this splint; however, any of the plastic-based materials would have been suitable. The stretch characteristic of the material was used to create the hole for the

Figure 4   The increase in the thumb index web span subsequent to serial static splinting and active exercise.

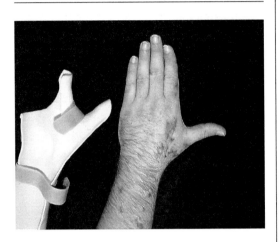

thumb in the hand component and intimate contour along the forearm. The outrigger was made of 3.2 mm brass welding rod, the traction unit combined nylon line and 3.2 mm Mercery thread, with anchorage to both hand and forearm components of the splint by small dress hooks. The force applied via the low-profile outrigger had to overcome resistance offered by the weight of the hand, gravity and friction via the pulley before it achieved the desired goal of positioning the joint at end range. The splint was worn for a minimum of 3 hours per day during a period when hand function was not required.

Supination was considered the more critical forearm range to gain for both self-care and vocational activities. Initially active range was 0°–19°. A serial progressive splint was applied for a period of 3 hours per day (Figure 14a in Chapter 4). This splint was chosen over a preformed splint because of availability and cost, and over a dynamic splint for its ease of fabrication and application. The fact that the force applied by the serial progressive design would remain constant to a range of motion was also considered an advantage over

the dynamic splint, which would continue to apply force once the tissues reached their maximum length. Therapists' experience suggests that tolerance to serial progressive traction is greater than dynamic traction, particularly where there is discomfort at end range on joint mobilization.

The wrist component only required the addition of anchorage Velcro® for the rotation straps. The elbow component of this splint was made from 3 mm Orfit® Classic. This material was chosen because the wrist component had been made of Orfit®, because it would adhere to the limb once activated, thus increasing the ease of managing a large piece of splinting material by eliminating the need to bandage, and because the strength of the material, combined with contour, would address the forces created by both the limb and the traction.

On initial application of this splint, just sustaining a position of several degrees supination was uncomfortable after 1 hour. Tolerance to the splint was gradually increased in half-hour increments over a week. Ultimately, Peter tolerated the splint for 3 hours, and was able to adjust the end range position several times over the period of wear.

Strength of wrist musculature was addressed in isolation using concentric and isometric exercises. Use of extensor digitorum communis to extend the wrist was discouraged. Strength in opposition of the thumb and flexion of the fingers were addressed using functional tasks and exercise putty.

After 6 weeks of intervention, active wrist range of motion had increased to 0°–17° extension (Figure 5), 0°–41° flexion, with forearm motion 0°–90° pronation and 0°–41° supination. Passive range was between 5° and 10° degrees higher. Pain was evident at the end range of all wrist motions, and during attempts at strong gross grip.

Figure 5   Deficit in active extension of the left wrist.

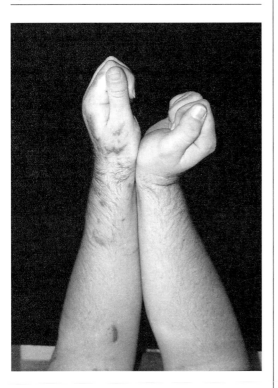

PHASE 3 (WEEK 18): STRENGTHENING PROGRAMME

An intensive 1-week period of therapy educated Peter in exercises to strengthen his left upper limb musculature. The programme included the need to undertake 'warm up' exercises prior to initiating more rigorous strengthening exercises using weights and vocationally based activities. Load, repetition and duration were manipulated to increase the stress applied to musculature gradually. Having attempted some mechanical repairs to his own car, Peter identified the need for greater wrist extension strength to maintain a neutral position during strong gross grip. Peter returned to part-time work at 22 weeks and full-time work at 25 weeks post-injury. Liaison with the vocational rehabilitation officer and employer deter-

mined restrictions on the maximum weight that he was able to lift. Modification to work practices were necessary to accommodate for the reduction in both strength and range, and the inability to take weight owing to pain when compression forces were transmitted through the wrist.

Hardening and strengthening of the left upper limb were achieved by participation in greater numbers of vocational and avocational tasks.

As range of motion in wrist extension plateaued at 0°–25°, dynamic wrist splinting ceased. Slow gains continued to be made in supination with the splint worn for 3 hours per evening until 25 weeks post-injury.

Summary

This case highlights the significant value splinting has in the management of musculoskeletal trauma. It also demonstrates that, where intensive therapy is not possible, and the patient is motivated and able to assume responsibility for intervention, provision of appropriate splints and a structured home programme can be very effective in facilitating the desired goal of recovery of function.

Case 2: Mrs Burke – Rheumatoid Arthritis (Post-MCP Arthroplasty Surgery)

The Person

Mrs Burke is a 69-year-old woman who was widowed 9 years ago. She has a married daughter with whom she shares a close and mutually beneficial relationship. Mrs Burke continues to live by herself in her own home unit where she cares for herself independently. Her daughter assists with heavy housework.

The Problem

Mrs Burke was diagnosed with rheumatoid arthritis (RA) 23 years ago. She has a progressive form of RA, and while there have been no major disease exacerbations, there has been a slow increase in insidious disease activity. Pharmacological management consisted of non-steroidal anti-inflammatory drugs (NSAIDs) for 15 years, and steroid therapy for 5–6 years. More recently, Mrs Burke has been managed with gold therapy.

All joints of the upper limbs are involved, with the shoulders and the MCP joints most affected. Moderate instability and loss of ROM is present in the shoulders. There is mild instability in the elbows, and the right wrist is very unstable with volar subluxation of the proximal carpals. Moderate ulnar deviation and volar subluxation was present at the MCP joints bilaterally (right worse than left). MCP arthroplasty (index to little finger) was performed on the right hand 2½ years ago with good result. The thumbs and fingers have good position and movement. The MCP deformities are in the form of fibrous ankylosis. Pain has never been a significant feature of the disease for Mrs Burke but, over the last 2 years, pain has been increasing to the point of affecting function, and radial peri-articular structures are stretching and loosening, with simultaneous shortening of ulnar and volar peri-articular structures. The extensor digitorum (ED) tendons are subluxed into the ulnar valleys at the MCPs. There is subsequent loss of passive and active ROM at the MCPs, with Mrs Burke reporting her major problem other than pain as 'weakness' in her hands, referring to her decreasing ability to grasp, manipulate and release objects.

MCP arthroplasty was performed on all fingers in the left hand. Surgery involved release of the tight ulnar and volar structures, tendon release of the ulnar intrinsics, insertion of the protheses, reconstruction of the radial collateral ligaments, and realignment of the ED and the extensor mechanism. A good ROM was achieved in surgery.

PATIENT'S OBJECTIVES

1. To regain hand function.
2. To reduce pain.
3. To maintain the level of ability in personal care and home duties.
4. To maintain the level of activity and enjoyment in leisure and social activities.

THERAPIST'S OBJECTIVES

To impact upon the tissue-healing process is the primary objective, aiming to maintain the elongation of joint volar and ulnar structures, and shortening of the dorsal and radial structures, which was achieved surgically. With this focus, the following objectives can be achieved:

1. Stability at the MCPs.
2. MCP joint mobility – passive and active ROM in the flexion–extension range.
3. Functionally pain-free MCPs.
4. Improved hand function.
5. Protection of repaired and other upper limb tissues bilaterally.
6. Maintenance of occupational performance status.

The Reasoning Process

Recovery from the arthroplasty surgery is considered in three phases – the acute inflammatory stage, the repair stage and the return to function stage. Each stage is longer than that identified in 'normal' tissue-healing stages owing to the slower healing rate.

CRITICAL ISSUES AFFECTING THE CLINICAL REASONING PROCESS

In determining the course of therapeutic intervention, consideration was given to:

1. RA is a chronic lifetime disease, which involves other tissues throughout the body. The disease compromises tissue integrity and healing.
2. Steroid therapy slows tissue healing and renders epithelial tissue fragile.
3. Mrs Burke is only able to be independent because of bilateral upper limb (UL) function.
4. Unilateral UL function will place unacceptable additional stress on the tissues of that limb and place them at risk of injury.
5. Mrs Burke is well motivated.
6. Support systems can be negotiated for and are acceptable for Mrs Burke on a short-term basis to assist with demanding daily self-care, household and gardening tasks.
7. Pre-existing deformity — the pathology and process that caused the deformity is still active and is likely to cause redeformation. Tissues have for many years been functioning abnormally. Following re-establishment of normal alignment physiological and cognitive retraining is required.

ACUTE INFLAMMATORY STAGE

The acute inflammatory stage extends for approximately 1 week, during which the critical feature is the protection of repaired structures. Management of cardinal signs of inflammation is the primary objective of therapy.

Problems, therapy options and splinting choice

1. Newly repaired, acutely inflamed tissues require protection from internal and external stressors. Therapy options are rest and immobilization by plaster, voluminous bandaging or splinting. Immobilization in a resting splint was chosen.
2. Post-operative oedema can be managed with elevation, ice, compression or immobilization. All modalities were utilized, given the importance of reducing the oedema quickly to prevent avoidable complications. Coban was used for compression, and immobilization was achieved with a resting splint.
3. Post-operative and inflammatory disease pain impedes participation in the therapy process and should be addressed as effectively as possible. Thermal modalities, compression and immobilization contribute to pain management. All modalities were utilized, again with immobilization by resting splint.
4. Absent hand function was unable to be impacted on as protection of repaired structures takes priority. Education regarding protection requirements was continuous throughout the therapy process. Recommendations and assistance addressing unilateral upper limb function for the uninvolved hand was continuous.

Splinting alternatives and rationale Application of a resting splint was identified as the most convenient and effective method to achieve immobilization. The prescribed position is ensured and not dependent on the person applying the modality. Wound care and dressings are unimpeded — in fact the splint enhances this procedure by maintaining the position required. A splint is the easiest immobilization modality to apply by the team caring for the patient.

The volar design is suitable because it allows protection of the suture line, it allows nursing access to the wound without risking position and it provides optimal support to repaired tissues against gravity. The position required to impact on repairing tissues was identified utilizing knowledge of anatomy and the surgical procedure. Wrist — extension of 20°, slight ulnar deviation; MCPs — 10° flexion, slight radial deviation (to maintain repaired extensor mechanism and radial collateral ligaments in a shortened position); preservation of transverse and oblique arches; IPs flexed approximately 20°. The resting splint was worn for 24 hours a day for the first week to achieve the primary objective of protection of repaired structures.

The desired features of the splint are for the material to be lightweight, to breathe for comfort and the protection of fragile skin, to be strong to maintain the prescribed position and to be easily moulded to avoid painful handling. Hexcelite® was the prescribed option, and it was contoured and reinforced to provide the desired strength. Straps were designed to be double normal width and made from soft Betapile™ to diminish pressure and prevent compromising circulation in the presence of oedema.

Occupational performance considerations During the acute inflammatory stage, unilateral hand function was prescribed for ADL, work and leisure. As this risked overstressing the tissues of the left hand, education was provided and reinforced continuously on risk factors and methods of protection. Support systems were identified and organized in preparation for return home.

REPAIR STAGE

The repair stage is characterized by the commencement of protected mobilization. The primary objective is to impact on the fibroplastic and maturation stages of wound healing to produce mobile and stable MCP joints. The repair stage lasts for approximately 6 weeks.

Problems, therapy options and splinting choice
1. Healing structures require continued protection from stressors. Therapy options include immobilization, restricted passive mobilization or restricted active mobilization. Restricted active mobilization with dynamic splinting was chosen (Figure 6). Resting splint was continued at night. Dynamic splinting provides protection from unwanted forces (MCP abduction and ulnar deviation) while permitting active flexion and extension.
2. During fibroplasia and maturation phases of wound healing, structures will adhere and the wound contract. Remodelling is required to maintain elongation of volar and dorsal capsular structures and shortening of the radial capsular structures. Active mobilization, initially in the dynamic splint will influence this remodelling.
3. Diminished passive ROM in the MCPs in flexion and extension can be addressed with passive mobilization (by therapist, by patient, by continuous passive motion machine), active mobilization (active or active assistive) or by mobilization with maximization of total end range time (TERT). Passive mobilization was performed twice daily. The splint allowed active flexion prescribed in therapeutic doses. At 5 weeks a flexion outrigger was added to the dynamic splint to provided TERT into flexion as passive flexion was being gained more slowly than desired.

Figure 6   Volar and dorsal views of a dynamic splint applied post-MCP arthroplasty surgery. Traction is applied in the directions of flexion and extension.

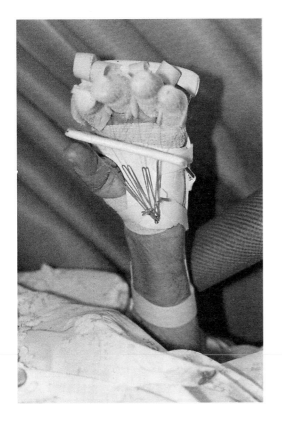 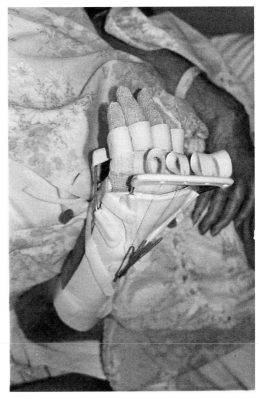

4. Active MCP extension was poor as pre-surgical deformity precluded normal extensor digitorum function. Post-surgically, the realigned extensor mechanism required protection and ED required retraining. Active or active–assistive mobilization could address this problem. Active–assistive mobilization in a dynamic splint was chosen as it provided the necessary protection and assistance to the repaired structures. From week 4 active extension mobilization was commenced.

5. Active MCP flexion required little intervention, given that pre-surgically this function was fair.

However, as ulnar intrinsics were released surgically, splinting is needed to impact on tissue healing to model fibroplasia and contraction. The dynamic splint provided this, allowing active flexion in prescribed doses. Active flexion was impeded by slow recovery of passive ROM in the later parts of the repair stage, which was addressed with a dynamic flexion component.

Splinting alternatives and rationale Dynamic extension splinting is the best option to impact on tissue healing and remodelling. Mobilization in the splint is more effective than passive mobilization in addressing adhesion formation, and is safer than unrestricted and unassisted active mobilization. The splint was prescribed to be worn as much as could be tolerated, beginning with 2 hours a day, building up to all day and some of the night by the end of week 1. The resting splint was worn for the remainder of the day. This regime provided maximal impact on tissue repair and return of function. For the first 3 weeks the splints remained on all the time and therapy was completed in the dynamic splint in order to provide maximum protection to the healing structures. In the second 3 weeks the dynamic splint was removed for twice-daily therapy.

The dorsal design of the dynamic MCP extension splint described in Chapter 6 required no modification. The splint covered the suture line so diligent wound care was required. An extended palmar bar was chosen to provide maximum support to the hand. The material needed to be highly drapable to ensure pain-free application and to achieve perfect contour to minimize pressure. Sansplint XR® was the material of choice. No lining was desired because remoulding, as oedema subsided, was required and linings pose a hygiene problem in the presence of wounds. Coban provided an interface between the splint and the skin with the advantage of adding compression for oedema management. A low-profile outrigger was chosen as this was the least bulky and cumbersome for Mrs Burke, and provided the length of base required to attach the prescribed 200 g force from the dynamic component. Finger cuffs were made from suede to provide comfort and durability.

Occupational performance considerations Mrs Burke was discharged from hospital in the second week. She attended the hand clinic as an outpatient for therapy and was able to be instructed on performing home therapy from week 3. During the first 3 weeks of the repair stage, function had to remain unilateral to achieve priority objectives. Education continued. From week 4, graded occupational performance activities commenced in the dynamic splint.

RETURN-TO-FUNCTION STAGE

The focus of this stage was graded reintroduction to functional use of the hand. Most wound repair activity occurs in the first 3 months and, therefore, this is when therapy can have the most impact. Protection of the repaired joints during function is a priority at this stage. The therapy of the previous stages was continued, reducing the passive and assistive aspects and increasing the active aspects.

Problems, therapy options and splinting choice

1. Mobility in MCP flexion and extension could be addressed by passive mobilization, active mobilization, active–assistive mobilization, maximizing TERT or functional use of the hand. A combination of all these modalities was used, with increasing emphasis on active and active functional mobilization. The gradation of activities that could be performed in the dynamic splint was increased, and performing specified activities without the splint commenced.

2. Stability of the joints and peri-articular structures remains an issue for the rest of Mrs Burke's life. Abduction, ulnar deviation and forced flexion of the MCPs are contraindicated, so activities must be analysed for stressors, which may produce these positions. The resting splint was prescribed for night-time use for a

year. Mrs Burke continues to wear the splint as she feels it is still beneficial. The dynamic splint with flexion and extension forces was used for periods of rest or no hand activity each day to continue impacting on the healing process. It was increasingly removed for safe, graded activities after 3 months, it was only used for very stressful tasks. An ulnar deviation protection splint was prescribed to be used for any activity that applies contraindicated stressors to the MCPs.

3. Pain-free, functional use of the hand was achieved. The strength of active MCP flexion and extension, required for functional activities, was achieved by a graded active–resistive therapy programme.

Splinting alternatives and rationale The ulnar deviation protection splint is a hand-based splint that does not impede function at any joint other than the MCPs. As the repaired structures are not able to resist severe contraindicated stressors, they are at risk of redeforming. The ulnar deviation protection splint allows continued function and mobility of the hand, but opposes the unwanted stressors to maintain the alignment of the MCPs.

Orfit® was chosen as it gives good contour for pressure distribution, and easy and pain-free application, and is strong when contoured. It is readily remoulded as hand and finger positions change. The splint was not lined as it is a working splint.

Occupational performance considerations Mrs Burke was able to increase bilateral function until, at 3 months, she had surpassed her previous independence status with a more mobile and pain-free left hand. She continued to protect the hand from contraindicated stressors, following therapeutic education and advice. She was able to manage occupational performance tasks with the level of assistance she was receiving prior to surgery.

Summary

Mrs Burke was discharged from therapy at 3 months. Active range of motion at the MCPs was 15°–70°. Finger position and rotation was good, and pain in the MCPs was minimal. The functional results of the surgery and therapy indicate that all critical issues of reasoning were addressed in designing the intervention programme.

Case 3: Mark – Neurological Dysfunction

The Person

Mark is 14-year-old boy who sustained a closed head injury as a result of a cycling accident at the age of 6. Mark lives with his parents, and a younger sister and brother. He attends the local high school. The majority of his academic subjects are undertaken through the education support unit with options in mainstream classes. He enjoys fishing and following his football team.

The Problem

Mark's diagnosis is spastic hemiplegia, affecting his right side. Mild tonal issues are evident in the left upper limb, but only when Mark is under considerable stress, at either physical or cognitive levels, or very tired. Prior to the injury, Mark was right dominant. He is ambulant but the presence of mild tonal patterns in his trunk, pelvis and hip contribute to a stable asymmetrical walking posture. The trunk tends to be laterally flexed to the right; however, all trunk movements have normal ROM. The tonal pattern in the right upper limb results in shoulder girdle protraction, shoulder internal rotation and extension, elbow flexion and forearm pronation. Active motion is limited in shoulder elevation and external rotation, elbow extension and supination greater than neutral.

Tone in the hand results in a pattern of moderate wrist flexion, with active wrist and finger extension (Pattern 2 described in Chapter 8). The tonal pattern present when undertaking specific tasks is more severe than that evident when simply moving the limb to the therapist's instructions. The thumb is adducted at the CMC joint. Flexion of the thumb MCP joint is simultaneous with finger flexion so pinch is inefficient.

Passive motion is limited at end range of shoulder external rotation. Contracture is present in the thumb index webspace, and in flexor digitorum profundus evidenced by an inability to extend the wrist and fingers simultaneously.

CLIENT'S OBJECTIVES

Increasing demands for academic performance at high school have highlighted the inefficiency of the right hand for assistive grasp and stabilization. Mark was not participating in regular therapy, and was encouraged to attend the clinic by his mother and schoolteacher who felt some form of splint to position the wrist and thumb was necessary. Mark did identify the fact that his wrist was tighter following a recent growth spurt, but was not enthusiastic about splinting. He indicated he had worn splints in the past and was not prepared to wear something that was big and ugly, or something that decreased the current use of his hand. He conceded he would consider options for intervention if they focused specifically on improving his performance in school-based activities. The

factors he identified were weakness in grip and inability to bring the thumb out of the palm during grasp, and difficulty supinating the forearm when carrying and reaching for objects.

THERAPIST'S OBJECTIVES

The facilitation of the efficient use of the right hand using interventions compatible with Mark's vocational requirements was the therapist's primary objective. The second objective was to provide Mark, his parents and teacher with information on the various options for intervention so that an informed choice could be made.

The Process

The evaluation of the upper limb was undertaken in a variety of postures in several challenging physical as well as cognitive tasks. It was important to determine how patterns of spasticity changed with intentional movement as this would have implications to splinting options. Performance in occupational specific tasks was videotaped as a measure of performance prior to intervention.

Options for splinting intervention were discussed with Mark and his mother. These included:

1. Doing nothing. The advantage of no intervention — no compromise to current patterns of hand and upper limb use, and no stresses for the family to enforce compliance to splinting intervention. The disadvantages are less tangible but pertain to a perspective of progression of the deformity and contracture with growth, and the persistence of inefficient patterns of hand use. These factors were raised taking a long-term perspective of how hand deformity and dysfunction can change with growth and age. In addition, the requirements of hand

function of an adult are often quite different from those of a child.

2. Addressing the thumb alone. If the thumb was stabilized in a position of abduction at the CMC joint and extension of the MCP joint, it would be in a better position for opposition to the fingers to assist grasp and pinch. Current ability to move the wrist and fingers would not be affected. Soft splinting was eliminated as an option as there is insufficient strength in the materials and design to achieve appropriate positioning during functional performance for a person of Mark's size and strength of tonal pattern. Thermoplastic splinting alternatives could position the thumb; however, the compromise of motion was identified as a limitation. The CMC/MCP spiral immobilization splint design was recommended as it covers a relatively small area of the palm leaving the wrist and finger function unimpeded. The splint would be applied and removed according to performance of those tasks where thumb stability or mobility was required.

As the client's objectives pertained to functional performance, splinting to address contracture in the webspace was not considered a high priority.

3. Addressing the wrist and thumb via some form of splinting. During intentional movement, the pattern of wrist flexion increased; however, Mark was able to flex and extend his wrist actively. For this reason, immobilization of the wrist using thermoplastic splinting intervention would be inappropriate. A dynamic Lycra® wrist gauntlet splint has the flexibility to allow movement of the wrist through mid-range with boning on the palmar surface restricting maximal wrist flexion and extension. Rotation of the thumb, with stability provided by boning, would facilitate functional grip and pinch. This splint would be primarily worn in the classroom to enhance hand posture for stabilization and grip.

4. Addressing the tonal pattern of the elbow and forearm. It was acknowledged that to address hand function effectively the stability and mobility of the rest of the upper limb had to be considered. The identified limitations in elbow extension forearm supination could be addressed by a supination extension arm sleeve splint. This dynamic Lycra®-based splint could be worn by itself or in combination with other forms of splinting intervention. The arm sleeve splint would be worn all day under the school uniform, and would not be visible if long sleeves were worn. The limitation of this intervention was the heat associated with wear during the hot summer months.

5. Other suggestions from family and teacher. Mark's mother indicated that her other son wore wrist gauntlets whilst roller skating and wondered whether a support of that nature would be suitable. Mark had tried one at home and found it held his wrist and he did not mind the appearance. The therapist suggested that the lack of custom fit and potential to move the wrist in the splint may present a problem when undertaking the finer tasks required at school. Modification of a commercial roller blading gauntlet was added to the list of options for consideration.

Several factors contributed to a risk of Mark's non-compliance. These were:

- His age and his desire to look similar his friends.
- His past experience with splinting intervention.
- His life disability with multiple facets that did not just involve his hand and upper limb.
- His mother and schoolteacher identified the need for splinting intervention and not Mark.
- The fact that Mark was not participating in

regular therapy and that monitoring of a multi-faceted splinting programme would occur at intervals of several weeks.

For these reasons Mark was given a week to decide which intervention he considered appropriate. On return to the clinic, he decided he really needed a more effective position for his thumb but was not prepared to have a splint on his wrist. Therefore, he chose the thermoplastic splint for his thumb. As the arm sleeve was not visible under his school uniform, Mark indicated he was prepared to 'give it a go'.

SPLINTING INTERVENTION

Following application of a supination extension arm sleeve splint, the resting posture of Mark's right upper limb was more extended at the elbow. Splints were gradually introduced for periods of several hours in the first week building up to wearing the splint all day at school. Over the following months of splint wearing, of approximately 6 hours per day, the range of active supination increased to approximately 40°. He indicated supination action did not feel so 'tight'.

Positioning the thumb in abduction at the CMC joint and slight flexion of the MCP improved grip and pinch. It was worn during performance of specific fine motor tasks.

OCCUPATIONAL PERFORMANCE OUTCOMES

Splinting focused to the specific occupational performance tasks identified by the client, which enabled him to determine the success of intervention. Mark continued to wear his splints as he was able to discern a difference in his skill performance not only in school-based activities but also in avocational tasks. Discarding splints during school holidays offered the opportunity to determine the ongoing value of intervention.

Summary

A splint of the very best design and manufactured with excellent workmanship is of no value unless it is worn by the client. Prescription of splints to meet the client's specific objective is paramount to compliance. This case study not only highlights issues pertaining to splinting to maximize compliance, but how splints of varying styles can be combined to facilitate occupational performance objectives.

Case 4: Sue – Cumulative Trauma (De Quervain's Syndrome)

The Person

Sue is 33 years old, and married with a 6-year-old daughter and 3-year-old son. She works part-time as a primary schoolteacher. Her husband is also a primary teacher, and is helpful and supportive. Sue has a network of family and friends who can provide occasional assistance in child minding.

The Problem

Two weeks prior to therapy contact, Sue experienced discomfort in her right (dominant) wrist and thumb following an extended period of writing on the blackboard with chalk. This discomfort was aggravated in the following days by picking up her son and further board-writing activities. The intermittent discomfort became constant pain during activities (especially childcare, driving and meal preparation) and was disturbing sleep. She had not previously experienced any problems with her hands. Sue referred herself to the hand clinic for advice. On examination, the tendons of abductor pollicis longus (APL) and extensor pollicis brevis (EPB) were palpably inflamed. The activities that triggered the injury placed an unacceptable active load on the involved muscles and tendons. The tissues were unable to respond normally to these stressors as the nature of the activity was resistive, repetitive and of extended duration with little recovery time. Additionally, the trigger activities placed the musculo-tendinous units at risk of exacerbation with inflammation.

PATIENT'S OBJECTIVES

1. To be free of pain.
2. To be able to carry out normal mothering, household and work duties.
3. To prevent recurrence of the injury.

THERAPIST'S OBJECTIVES

1. To facilitate resolution of inflammation.
2. To protect susceptible tissues from re-injury throughout the recovery period.
3. To educate the patient on the nature, management and prevention of the injury.
4. To achieve return to full function with modification of activities which predispose tissues to cumulative trauma.

The Reasoning Process

Recovery from De Quervain's tenosynovitis is considered in three phases – the acute/subacute inflammatory stage, the weaning-off stage and the function-with-protection stage.

CRITICAL ISSUES AFFECTING CLINICAL REASONING PROCESS

1. The rate of recovery is impeded by the nature of the insult, which contributed to the injury. The first step in the management of inflammation is to remove the primary 'noxious' agent to allow healing to occur. This is difficult as hand activity will irritate the condition.
2. Modification or avoidance of activities is difficult in the presence of the demands of motherhood and vocational expectations.
3. Sue is otherwise healthy. She is intelligent and highly motivated, and is supported by a caring family.
4. Therapy consists of splint prescription and application only. Sue does not return for regular weekly therapeutic intervention, so full understanding of the requirements of management is essential.

ACUTE/SUBACUTE INFLAMMATORY STAGE

This stage can extend for up to 6 weeks, during which the focus of management is on protection of the injured structures. Pain and loss of function are features of this stage. Inflammation is subacute but the healing tissues tolerate less stress before subsequent re-injury. Recurrent re-injury threatens to create a chronic condition.

Problems, therapy options and splinting choice The management of inflammation can be achieved through ice, elevation, electrotherapeutic agents, or immobilization. The first three modalities are intermittent, which is unacceptable in the light of the pathology. They are inconvenient because of the unpredictable nature of mothering responsibilities, and they require taking little responsibility for one's recovery because of their passive nature. Compression garments are contraindicated as Sue constantly has her hands in water for mothering and work tasks. Immobilization of the structures in a working splint was prescribed.

Splinting alternatives and rationale A radial thumb wrist immobilization splint (Figures 9 and 10 in Chapter 7) achieved the desired immobilization of the injured structures, while allowing freedom on the ulnar side for mobility, sensation and function. The position of immobilization addressed all the joints crossed by the structures and placed them at minimal tension. The wrist was in neutral deviation and 20° extension. The carpometacarpal (CMC) joint was slightly abducted and extended, and the MCP joint was flexed only to the degree that allowed thumb to index pinch. The IP joint was not involved as the structures do not impact at that joint.

The material chosen was Sansplint XR® (Polyflex®) for its ease of application and rigidity. No lining material was added as the splint was to be used in water.

The splint was worn 24 hours a day for this stage, to be removed only for bathing or if Sue was in restful activity. The objective of the splint was to prevent stressors of the tissues having an effect. The tissues must not be stretched (either by active flexion of the thumb or by position of the wrist and hand). Active contraction of APL and EPB is minimized. This allowed for reduction in the inflammatory process and diminishing of the pain.

Occupational performance considerations Although the splint prevents stretch of APL and EPB, active contraction during activities of daily living can still occur, and would be resisted by the splint, placing these structures at risk of re-

inflammation. Education of appropriate hand activity was provided to prevent this occurring.

WEANING-OFF STAGE

In this stage the evidence of acute inflammation and pain has diminished, with the hand pain-free at rest. Risk of re-injury remains acute for approximately 3 months.

Problems, therapy options and splinting choice A programme of weaning off the splint to allow return of mobility without injury was undertaken. Therapy options of passive or active mobilization with the range of therapeutic modalities available was not considered appropriate given Sue's daily commitments. Mobilization was successfully incorporated as part of normal ADL, causing minimal disruption and loss of time.

Splinting alternatives and rationale The splint was worn extensively at first with removal for rest periods only. Analysis of ADL was undertaken to identify potential stressors of stretch or active contraction of APL/EPB. The splint was applied for all identified activities.

Occupational performance considerations Those activities which provided active mobilization within safe ranges (avoiding extremes of flexion and extension) had no component of resistance and were not excessively repetitive were introduced without the splint on a gradual scale. Activity was prescribed to provide increasing mobilization at regular intervals through the day with the splint being worn for the remainder to continue protection. The focus of this stage was on Sue being able to identify risks, read warning signs, and self-evaluate and modify activity.

FUNCTION-WITH-PROTECTION STAGE

Recovery is completed but the tissues are now predisposed to re-injury. This stage extends for the whole future given that one's hands are rarely quiet for long. Educated use of the hands in daily function, with recognition of, and protection from, risk activities is the feature of this stage.

Problems, therapy options and splinting choice The objective is to maintain the mobility, strength and function the hand has achieved during the therapy process. Daily activities are used to achieve this and, in response, a maintained level of function improves performance in daily activities.

Splinting alternatives and rationale The splint was still able to be applied if Sue had concerns of re-inflammation. It rests and immobilizes painful inflamed tissues, but at this stage, it serves as a cognitive cue to limit stressors.

Occupational performance considerations Sue returned to full function at 3 months post-trauma, with care and protection from stressors that placed her APL / APB at risk. Sue occasionally experiences pain from activities but is able to identify and solve the problem before it re-injures her hand.

Summary

These four cases studies illustrate the vital role splinting has in the management of upper limb dysfunction. Each case study has focused on issues critical to the clinical reasoning process underpinning intervention that is designed to meet the specific objectives of the patient and therapist. Successful splinting intervention is dependent on appropriate prescription, design and fabrication by the therapist, and compliance to the wearing schedule on the part of the patient.

Index

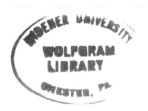